The Last Tango with

BUTTER

Everything your Grandmother knew
but didn't know how to explain

Melissa Putt RNC

Library and Archives Canada Cataloguing in Publication

CIP data on file with the National Library and Archives

ISBN 978-1-926582-71-9 Hard cover
ISBN 978-1-926582-72-6 Trade paperback

Dedicated to Lucy
'up to the moon and back'
Mommy

CONTENTS

INTRODUCTION

I wrote this book for several reasons. But if I had to narrow things down for simplicity's sake I would say this: I wrote this book to vent my frustration at the misinformation that abounds in the mainstream media about so many aspects of nutrition. Every day of my career as a nutritionist and fitness consultant I find myself struggling to convince people of their primal right to nourishment – that we do indeed 'have time' to eat real food, and digest it. This is a constant struggle, in the face of the hundred different flashy diets, processed, manufactured 'health foods', nutritionally senseless 'meal plans' and masochistic philosophies of self-denial that we're all exposed to in the course of a typical week.

Though it's a complicated business on the biochemical level, on a primal level nutrition can and should be intuitive. Health is not going to come from engineered foods that manufacturers hype with flashy advertisements and packaging. Food that's up to the job of building our bodies one cell at a time, and ensuring these cells perform their functions within healthy organs and systems, must be wholesome and come from all of nature's pure sources. Once they're given good raw material to work with, our bodies will do the rest, and build the best and strongest structure that we could ask for. We will age better, suffer less disease, and feel clearer in mind and body when all the building blocks fit together.

The past two generations of consumers have been led far astray from any natural relationship to nourishment, and our children will suffer as a consequence of our complex misunderstanding of what food is and what it's for. Their diseased bodies will age faster than we could have imagined, taxing our healthcare system and threatening our future as a productive society. With this book I hope to give parents a tool that will help them embrace a basic, and time-tested, sense of proper well-rounded nutrition, and help them recognise the dangers of stuffing their offspring with refined and manufactured food products dressed up with 'nutritional' additives to make them look healthy. I hope to help parents, and everyone else, recognise that it's a mistake to eliminate wholesome, natural foods because of perceived lack of time, or because of a belief that wonderful, forbidden fat-rich foods are not necessary for growth and development. I want to convince people that our own bodies are often wiser than nutritional science when it comes to knowing what constitutes a healthy diet.

My third reason for writing this book is to draw attention to a particularly serious example of the profound unwisdom that official nutritional policy so often embraces – in the form of a particular belief paradigm that's grown up over the last forty years. Following the advice of government officials, nutritional pseudo-science and mainstream media selling false hopes and illusory promises of health, the last two generations have consumed more omega 6 fatty acid than any other generation ever, anywhere in the world. These omega 6 oils from vegetable sources have systematically displaced saturated fats from animal sources from our diets. This fundamental dietary shift was supposed to secure a lifetime of health, free of disease and overweight. Today we live the results of those radical dietary changes, which were conceived and propagated without any proper scientific consensus. Yes omega 6 unsaturated oil is good for us, but not without the butter.

There are some rather complicated technical sections in this book explaining the metabolism of fats. Even if you disdain the dry science, try to read on and listen to the sense in the words. It is a story reflected through the wisdom of my dear Grams; for she intuitively ate well, even though she lived her adult life in the heart of an industrial union town. If she can do it with a grade six education and five children to feed, so can we.

CHAPTER 1

PRELUDE

When I was 19, and straight out of high school except for several months toiling in low paid jobs to save money, I set off on a solo cycling tour that took me through Western Europe and Morocco. I was hell-bent on getting somewhere in life, but I lacked the confidence to head straight off to university like all my closest friends had done. Somehow, being alone in strange countries where I didn't speak the language or understand the social rules and protocols seemed easier to face than the University of Western Ontario's big modern library, and another four years under my mother's roof. I was enamoured of foreign languages and far-off exotic places, and most of all in love with with the idea of adventure. The prospect of having to make important choices all on my own, and the thought of meeting people that hadn't grown up in a conservative Anglo-Saxon town, thrilled me to the point of taking action. I already spoke French fluently from short student exchanges, and I had competed intently at long distance running throughout high school; but beyond this I didn't really excel at much. So a physical adventure that took me through the relatively safe environs of Europe suited me well. I could test my body physically and drink up the music of foreign languages – playing to my strengths.

At the time I was fit, but not as strong as I would be in my late 20s and 30s; at about 120 pounds and 23% body fat, I was an average size for my 5 foot 3 inch frame. I already had a keen interest in nutrition, but I was still far more interested in adventure than in university. And my knowledge of what constituted a healthy diet was skewed by the misinformation served up by the media at the time – and in such large portions! Throughout the 1980s vegetarianism was seen as the only healthy and righteous way to live, and back then, just like so many teenage girls that I counsel today, I wouldn't even consider eating meat. Fruit on its own for breakfast was also all the rage. The popular nutrition and diet book

Fit for Life, by marketing giants Marilyn and Harvey Diamond, was a must-read at the time. Some things haven't changed much, and ideas about nutrition and health are still disseminated to a knowledge-hungry populace on much the same basis, with marketing savvy trumping the experience and reputation of professional health practitioners.

And so I found myself in Europe. On a typical day of my cycling adventure I would rise early, at six or seven AM, and start the morning with whatever hot beverage was served up in the region I happened to be in; this could be anything from milky coffee to strong black tea, from mint tea to hot double espresso. Then I'd hit the back roads for a tough 100- or 150-kilometre bicycle ride. At least once a week I'd cycle 200 to 250 kilometres in a day. The terrain in Europe is challenging, certainly compared to southwestern Ontario where I now live, and where I'd done some road riding and training to prepare for my tour. The day on which I started the morning at sea level, cycled to 2900 meters in the Pyrenees by noon, did a 1000 meter descent, then climbed back again to 2800 meters, wasn't all that unusual in the course of my tour. This is pretty demanding cycling under any conditions – even more so when you're carrying panniers loaded with 30 pounds of equipment and provisions. One entry in my journal describes a day I was in the saddle (as we aficionados call the bicycle seat) for 12 continuous hours, on a vertical climb against a ferocious headwind and hard rain; I was afraid to stop and dismount for fear of not being able to regain my momentum and re-establish a cadence.

Pyrenees, Pau France to Jaca Spain – 2888 meters; October, 1986. *"A misty rain fell as I climbed the 27 km incline for hours. And I can remember crying because of the physical pain that in some strange way satisfied me. "* (From my journal)

After I returned home, our local magazine and newspaper ran stories about my trip, which they seemed to feel made for a fascinating tale. At the time I thought everyone was exaggerating their interest in my adventures; I couldn't see what was so special about what I'd done. The reporters always grilled me as much about what I *ate* on my tour as about where I'd ventured and who I'd met, and members of local cycling groups did the same. Nutrition was clearly the focus of growing interest, and seen as a subject that called for self-education, especially among the 'athletic' types to whom I told my story. And as it happened, for the entire year I was away I had kept impeccable records of my grocery bills, in an effort to manage a strict budget of $5,000. These records in effect offered a detailed, day-to-day account of what I'd eaten on the trip.

Much of this money had been socked away from a cycling accident settlement. The rest was saved from toiling 11pm to 7am as a waitress in a pancake house, and then from 9am to 5pm teaching aerobics at Woody's Fitness in London Ontario. In the two-hour gap between jobs I used to sleep in the sauna at the fitness club. That $5000 hadn't fallen into my lap! And soon after I started my trip I began to carefully record all my purchases, including groceries. I rarely ate in a restaurant.

As it turned out, I sometimes ate pasta that I prepared in the kitchens of the hostels where I camped for the night. The pasta was always covered in "lots and lots of BUTTER." (This is me, quoted in Encounter Magazine, London, Ontario, October 3, 1987). At the time I had no idea of the significance of short, medium and long chain fats, or about how butter would protect my vulnerable intestines, or about how butter was metabolised like a source of carbohydrates. I just knew that it was salty, and it made me feel light enough to go out and pedal for hours the next day without ever having a too-full feeling in my belly.

I came to choose my foods on the basis of how well they made me feel during the day's cycling. In contrast to the magic of buttery pasta, eating pastries and cookies for lunch, which I sometimes did during the early part of my tour, left me feeling tired and drained, with dead legs. This, I learned years later in my nutrition and endocrinology classes, was based on severe fluctuations in my insulin levels, an overworked pancreas during sleep, and simply because overeating simple carbohydrates resulted in their being stored as triglycerides, since the glycogen stores of my exercising muscles were already replenished.

All the food I bought had to be kept, along with everything else I needed for the trip, in panniers hanging off the back of my bicycle. So I couldn't carry a wide variety of foods. And I had to make the best of the food I did carry; the heat inside my panniers would melt all but the hardest cheese, but instead of throwing the liquid cheesy mess away I would spread it onto bread, or dip a sweaty finger into it for a quick snack. Because I bought the food in stores, in retail quantities, I would usually end up eating the same thing for a couple of meals until it was all gone – and this pattern helped me recognize which foods made better fuels. At the time I only paid attention to how I felt, and couldn't have cared less about nutritional value. I just wanted the energy to cycle hard and strong every single day.

"October 20, 1986. That's the date I rode out of Spain into Portugal and I felt it would be forever. I can remember having several pesos in change. The departure felt so permanent and anticipated. I celebrated by spending all the loose change in a little tuck shop on the boarder. I felt like a rich girl when I bought my treats and the clerk kept giving me change. So I kept buying treats until all the coins were spent. I ate cookies, chocolate, and pastries until it was obvious my eyes were way bigger than my belly." (From my journal))

I didn't know it at the time, but this system of trial and error actually amounted to an important, if informal, experiment in nutrition and endurance exercise. My records show that the foods I purchased most often were butter, cheese, yoghurt, sardines, fruit, and pasta. Despite my twelve-hour days on the road, pastas and pastries were the least significant part of my diet. This pattern of eating was (and still is) contrary to current nutrition wisdom for endurance sports. But pasta had to be prepared in a hostel kitchen, at the end of a long day's cycling, so by default I ate less of it. I did eat lots of bread – which I used as a platform for the wonderful variety of fresh cheeses. When I was on the coast, sardines could usually be bought from the fishermen on the beach and eaten right off the skewer; and canned sardines could always be found when I was cycling further inland. Pastries were an exciting novelty for a few weeks, until I got deathly ill on almond-paste croissants in Antwerp, Belgium. I vomited and defecated my way to 100 pounds in a single week, and I wouldn't touch anything containing almond paste for a good ten years. The owner of the travellers' hotel would knock on my door every morning to collect the $12.00 for my room, and to see if I had died and freed it up entirely. Oh, and the bathroom was down the hall, and shared with the occupants of six other rooms.

Travelling alone, I was very often invited into the homes of locals. Despite the language barrier in Spain and Portugal, families were intrigued by my adventures and invited me in to taste their wine, food, and gracious hospitality. I am sure now, as a mother myself, that they wouldn't have wanted their own daughters to cycle through Europe and Morocco alone, but they were genuinely curious about *my* travels. My mother had sewn Canadian flags on every pair of my cycling shorts, and this proved to be a passport into the lives and culture of the Europeans. When I rode into a town where I intended to stay for the night, I would try to orient myself quickly regarding all the necessities: grocery store, pensions or inexpensive family-run hotels, and local maps. If the town was small, news of the arrival of a solo female 'Canadian' cyclist would spread like wildfire. It often felt as if the whole population had come out to greet me. There was often cheering, especially when they knew that I had climbed several mountains peaks to reach their town – like in Rhonda Spain at close to 2000 meters. I quickly learned what the phrase "Yea Chica" meant.

It was these spontaneous interactions that put me in direct contact with the local inhabitants. The mothers would come out with cold water and ripe tomatoes and figs, so plump and luscious, and hand them to me as I pushed my bike slowly through the town trying to orient myself and find a place to rest. Shopkeepers often made a quick phone call, and in no time a family would appear and extend an invitation for me to stay in their home. It happened so often, and I cherish those moments with welcoming strangers as one of the most important memories of my journey. And their loving preparation of the meals we shared told me everything I failed to interpret from each new language that I struggled to learn. I would be given my own room and hot bath water, which was a treat, and the bed always had crisp sheets to sleep in. (I think this is because they hung the sheets out in the air to dry, then ironed them)

But best of all I got to sit at a family dinner table and eat the real local cuisine with gracious and generous hosts. And in every home I was invited into, in every country I travelled through, everyone was always so passionate about the food being served. Despite the language barrier, which was pretty profound at the beginning of my adventures, we always found a way to communicate the basic concepts. There was always a story about where the oil came from, or the exceptional flavour of the tomatoes that year, or the extra secret spice in the sausage.

As time passed and my Spanish and Portuguese improved, these late-night conversations (late-night because the Europeans eat very very late compared to North Americans, for whom this is one of those forbidden dietary practices) became a little easier to manage after long days drenched in hot sun and hundred-mile plus bike rides. And, well, frankly I didn't see, hear, or experience a hint of the Mediterranean diet, as we as North Americans have been led to believe it is practised. Yes they used olive oil, but there was absolutely no abstinence – no lack of meat or dairy or saturated fat. The Europeans prepared food in ways quite different from those I'd known growing up. They cooked it differently; they added more flavour and spice; they drank more wine; they sat longer with more people at their meals. But they ate meat, eggs, cheese, and butter.

> "Braga Portugal. November, 1986. *"In the living quarters there was no stove, no fridge, no tiled counter tops. This was the Portuguese way of life. They preferred it to the modern, sleek, fully equipped kitchen upstairs. Flies were everywhere, and the wooden table was filled with typical Portuguese food: bread made with cornmeal, ground the previous day, fried eggs, fried potatoes, and thick slabs of meat. How would I tell them I didn't eat meat? The mother cooked over the open pit fire. The basement had a winery filled with kegs of wine left to mature. The grapes came from their own land, as did the wheat that was the flour, the plum that was the prune, the herbs that were dried to spice. "* (From my journal)

It seems fair to declare that my endurance efforts were not fuelled by 60%-70% carbohydrates, as all the sports nutrition manuals have been recommending they should be for the last 20 years. My efforts were fuelled by equal parts of carbohydrates, proteins, and above all, quality fats from oil, fish, meat, (I eventually recanted my oath of vegetarianism) cheese, and butter. As a kid straight out of high school I had stumbled, pretty much by accident, on nutritional principles that vested interests and well meaning authorities had worked together to drive out of people's collective memory across much of North American society.

CHAPTER 2

FULL FAT NUTRITION:
A THOROUGH PERSPECTIVE

Rehabilitating fat

For decades, dietary fat has been the public enemy number one of dieters and the health conscious, who have been convinced by the apparent scientific consensus concerning its detrimental role in human health. An entire new industry has emerged, dedicated to developing and marketing food products that enable us to systematically exclude fats from our diets. The marketing campaigns for 'fat free', 'low cholesterol' and 'light' foods have worked hard to persuade consumers that fat is a substance to be avoided at all costs, a belief that has been encouraged not just through direct argument, but by implication, through the very ubiquity of these ('healthy!' 'new!') products. And animal fats have been seen as worst of all. Foods that contained fat inherently and naturally – things like eggs, steak, and butter – have become substances prohibited to anyone seeking optimal health. Butter was banished and replaced with margarine made from unsaturated vegetable oils. Lard has long since disappeared from the pantry, and vegetable oil shortenings have been baked into our pies for forty years.

Dietary fat has been the single most important element in discussions about human nutrition since not long after the process of hydrogenation was patented in the 1920s. Since that milestone, fat has been modified, refined, and substituted right out of our diet. We have been a 'fat-phobic' society for over fifty years. But after decades of minimizing fat consumption, of completely modifying the natural composition of the fats we still eat, and of ignoring the human need for dietary fat, we are finally beginning to re-discover the truth: that fats are an essential component of human nutritional health.

The first step in the rehabilitation of fats, and in the growth of a more sophisticated understanding of what makes fats good or bad, came with recognition of the important role played by essential omega 3- and omega 6-rich oils, and by seeds and nuts, currently referred to collectively as 'good fats'. This knowledge insinuated its way up from cottage industries and health food stores into mainstream consumer consciousness and into the big grocery chain stores. Consumers, convinced for 40 years that there were good, concrete reasons to avoid all fats, finally got the nod of approval to eat nuts and seeds as nutritious and balanced snacks. And then, in early 2000, the detrimental effects of the modified trans fatty acids were suddenly big news in the mainstream media. The ensuing food policy changes forced manufacturers to abandon their use of the stable but deleterious trans fats, clearly the perfect example of a 'bad fat', if ever there was one.

Of course, any natural health practitioner, even twenty years ago, understood the downside to trans fats; none of it was new knowledge. Together, the growth of the internet and the determination of consumers looking for answers to questions about nutrition and health led to a widespread recognition of the harmful effects of this modified fat. Consumers and committed food scientists forced the hand of policy-makers, and they in turn curbed the use of trans fatty acids by the manufacturers of commercial food products.

Clarifying the Classification of Fats

The classification of fats as simply 'saturated', 'unsaturated' or monounsaturated' really is an inadequate basis for then judging their contribution to health or disease. It is oversimplified to the point of being misleading. All dietary fats and oils are made up of different combinations of *fatty acids*. The configuration of the carbon and hydrogen atoms out of which all fats are constructed, and the number and type of bonds holding everything together, determine how these constituent fatty acids are categorized – into monounsaturated, saturated, polyunsaturated, trans or conjugated fatty acids. The crude everyday classification above is simply based on the characteristics of the *dominant* fatty acid, ignoring the fact that there are other components in any oil or fat. Butter, for example, is made up of 14 different fatty acids, saturated *and* unsaturated.

The lazy and imprecise categorization of fats has created a problem for today's nutrition-conscious consumer, much as the oversimplification of carbohydrate classification created problems for the consumer from the 1970s until well into the 1990s. Nature produces all of these fats, even its own *natural* versions of the much maligned trans fats, and all of them can offer health benefits. The normalisation of this oversimplified classification of fats went hand in hand with the official policy that saturated fats in particular should be avoided or restricted. The truth, like the fats themselves, is more complicated; all natural fats offer benefits, but if eaten out of balance with one another, they can all have negative affects on health.

In my twenty years of practice as a nutritionist and exercise coach, I have never had a client who was not avoiding saturated fats. And nutritional authorities and food marketers have made no attempt to help the consumer distinguish between the *different* saturated fats, or to understand how each of these saturated fats can affect human health and metabolism. The oversimplification involved in lumping all saturated fats together in one functional category has encouraged people to avoid eating very healthy, necessary, and *nutritious* saturated fats. We need to understand the complexities of fat, and of the human need for fat, before we can make dietary choices that will optimise or enhance our health. How we fry with fats, how we extract fats from vegetable, nut and seed sources, and how much fat we eat, all contribute to the beneficial or harmful affects that fats can have on our health. It's curious that fats have had a bad reputation for so long, even though we *know* the vital, complex dependency our biology has on them. The oversimplification of fat biology, the generic guidelines for fat intake, and the rudimentary categorization of fats have (mis)led health-conscious consumers down the garden path towards potential health problems. *All* natural fats are essential to health, saturated fats included.

Being a saturated fat does not make you a bad food! We have to stop categorizing all saturated fats and fatty foods as equal, and as equally evil. Saturated fats are as different from one another as the foods that contain them. The components of fats and oils that are currently largely ignored in dietary recommendations might have very important influences on health and degenerative disease. Fats are more than just their 'fatty acid profiles', but the grouping of fats into oversimplified categories has prevented our recognising the importance of developing a more detailed understanding of their complex chemistry, and its meaning for our health. Fats have been judged, and vilified or promoted, solely on the basis of their saturation level rather than with an eye to their synergistic dependence upon each other – and it is this interdependence that determines whether/when/how fats are good or bad. It follows that achieving a proper *balance* of saturated to unsaturated fats is the essential nutritional goal, rather than the elimination or reduction of saturated fats and their substitution with unsaturated alternatives.

I believe that the next frontier for the nutrition-conscious consumer is a thorough understanding of saturated fats – an understanding that offers insight into the current dogma and helps us to move beyond it. The ideal of a diet purged of saturated fat has been the basis for so many promises of improved health and longevity; and the self evident hollowness of these promises, as people continue to suffer from the degenerative diseases that this diet was supposed to save us from, has motivated many consumers to search for their own answers once again.

I predict that the next 'essential fats' to grace our kitchens and restaurants will be the ones that were banished from healthy households 40 years ago. These essential saturated fats have been sorely missed in our diets and in the diets of our children. We were lured out of the arms of Mother Nature and into the clutches of food manufacturers who claimed to have established an authoritative science of nutritional health; but consumers are now aware of the poverty of the food industry's pretensions, and are seeking the truth themselves. The return to butter and saturated fats is imminent! The time has come to spread the word that the really important shift in human fat consumption, the change in eating habits that has done so much harm to human health, has not been an increasing consumption of saturated fat *but a growing dietary imbalance in the proportion of all the other dietary fats relative to saturated fat.*

My Grandma Doolittle was born in 1889. By 1909, when she was 19 years old, the average beef consumption in North America was 54 pounds per person per year. Cattle were still largely grazed on grass and clover, not fed corn and grain in feed lots as most are today; and what cattle are fed greatly affects the fatty acid profile of beef and dairy products. Heart disease at the time was relatively rare. Some researchers argue that this was in part because the testing modalities were not as advanced or as available as they are today, and that perhaps heart disease was more prevalent than the contemporary reports indicate. There was a high incidence of viral and bacterial infection in this pre-antibiotic era, leading to illnesses like rheumatic fever – which is known to damage the heart muscle and to contribute to heart disease. It is generally agreed that heart disease did increase between 1909 and 2000 by approximately 40%. As we'll see later in the book, the statistics available for the reported incidence of heart disease have been somewhat skewed as a result of changing nomenclature and testing modalities, and the reporting bias of death certificates. Nevertheless, the belief that heart disease, saturated fat and cholesterol are intimately related is not in question so far as mainstream health care is concerned, and this belief is still aggressively proselytised.

Beef consumption rose during this same period, 1909-2000, to 79 pounds per person per year. Since beef is high in saturated fat it made sense that beef consumption statistics would be used to give weight to the correlation between saturated fats and the heart disease epidemic. But consider the following facts: poultry consumption increased a whopping *288%* during the same period, from 18 to 70 pounds per person per year. My Grandma Doolittle didn't eat her chickens. She kept them for their high protein, life-sustaining (and cholesterol-rich!) eggs. Poultry is higher in unsaturated than saturated fats so its contribution to the heart disease epidemic was never considered.

And vegetable oil consumption has increased even more dramatically since 1909. My Grandma never used much oil; it wasn't available all year round back then. However, butter was. Grandma used butter, cream, and lard! 100 years ago, vegetable oils from corn, sunflower, safflower etc. were just getting their foot in the door, especially in cold climates like Canada's, and it wasn't until the 1920s that hydrogenated oils appeared in shortenings and margarines. There was no canola oil, as it had not yet been 'invented'. In the course of the 20th century North Americans' consumption of vegetable oils increased an astonishing 437%, from 11 to 59 pounds per person per year.

Can saturated fat really be the main culprit in the explosion of degenerative disease and heart failure among North Americans? Increased saturated fat consumption has certainly been blamed for the increase in disease, while other foods and food groups whose consumption has also increased over the past 100 years have been arbitrarily let off the hook. The only foods that are consumed in smaller quantities now than 100 years ago are butter, lard, tallow, vegetables and eggs. Consumption of lard, tallow and butter has dropped from 30 pounds to just under 10 pounds per person per year; North Americans are not consuming saturated fats in anything like the amounts we were at the turn of the century. Remember that butter, lard, and tallow are the purported enemies of modern health. Eggs were a staple of any healthy diet back then; now they are seen by many people as little better than poison.

Consumption of whole milk also declined in the course of the last century — by 50% — while the consumption of skim milk more than doubled. Fresh fruit (except citrus fruits), fresh vegetables, fresh potatoes, barley, millet, rye, and oats are eaten in smaller quantities today than a century ago, while consumption of sugar and other sweeteners such as corn syrup, honey, maple syrup, high fructose corn syrup, has increased dramatically. North American sugar consumption in 1909 averaged 4 pounds per person per annum, while the current intake is 60 pounds per year of sugar, *plus* 46 pounds of corn syrup. That totals a 4.6 oz daily habit of sweet stuff per person, year-round. And yet our heart disease epidemic is still blamed on our 'high saturated fat diet'! There are many factors that may have contributed to declining heart health, *but an increased consumption of saturated fat can't be one of them, because we're eating less saturated fat.*

Consumption patterns over the last century represent clear evidence that the saturated fat-heart disease hypothesis should be reopened for re-evaluation. Saturated fat has many essential metabolic functions in the body and comes from food sources that play a beneficial role in human health. While official food policy might take generations to change, an understanding of the nutritional importance of saturated fat can empower individuals to make their own dietary choices when it comes to the consumption of fat.

If there is a single category of food whose consumption has increased most rapidly in the last century, it is the 'modified' foods. Foods are now pasteurized, ultra pasteurized, pre-cooked, pre-packaged, preserved with chemical stabilizers, touched up with colour enhancers, irradiated, bleached, and reconstituted into food 'products'. We *are* eating more meat; but in light of all the other dramatic changes in our diets, should saturated fat be seen as even remotely connected to the health issues that have emerged over the last century? Modified whole foods such as skim milk do not contribute to human health as their natural predecessors did. Yet neither the modified fats in vegetable shortenings, vegetable oils and margarines, nor entirely processed foods like skim milk, processed cheeses and sweeteners, have ever been closely scrutinized for their possible detrimental affects on human health. The critical changes in the North American diet, during a century that has seen heart disease rise to epidemic proportions, continue to be ignored and negated. Perhaps the food policy-makers should get ready for the real food fight; we are now fighting to restore our health, and it is affected in many profound ways by the food we eat. Food policy must come to recognize the health consequences of cheap, pasteurized, modified, reconstituted foods, and at the same time acknowledge the benefits of wholesome non-processed, fresh foods, *even those rich in saturated fats.*

The First Vilification of Saturated Fats

The belief that unsaturated fats, and margarines made with them, would save the arteries of America was based in part on population studies done by Ancel Keys, who in the late 1950s travelled the world studying and recording a wide variety of traditional diets. Keys rightfully observed that the diets of the Mediterranean region were rich in unsaturated olive oil, and that the Japanese were eager consumers of fish – also high in unsaturated oil. He concluded that the cultures least affected by heart disease were those that did not eat saturated fat. And it followed from this, in his view, that it was saturated fat that was wreaking such havoc on the health of Americans. There are obvious shortcomings in Keys work, however. For example, the Masai people were excluded from Key's international comparison of diet and health. The diet of the Masai is based largely on fresh, unpasteurized cow's milk (rich in cream and cholesterol), and wild red meats. Their diet can be devoid of fibre and vegetables for seasons at a time. And yet the incidence of heart disease is negligible. Several other traditional diets heavily dependent on saturated fats were arbitrarily left out of the study.

Keys was a passionate researcher, with a strong and unyielding hypothesis that cholesterol and saturated fat constituted the root cause of heart disease. This became known as Ancel Key's 'lipid hypothesis' or 'diet-heart lipid hypothesis', and would serve as the theoretical basis for the perceived links between saturated fat, cholesterol, and heart disease that have played such a central role in shaping the modern North American diet. Ancel Keys passed away in February 2005 at 100 years of age, perhaps further supporting his anti-saturated fat theory. However, much to my disappointment he didn't donate his body to science, so that we could all have a good look at his polyunsaturated-rich arteries.

After his world travels of the late 1950s, much of Key's technical research took place in a laboratory setting that did not reflect the true diet or lifestyle of any human population. This laboratory research used methods involving extreme diet and nutrient control to isolate 'the' nutrient causing the rise in blood cholesterol and arteriosclerosis, and led to the launch of the famous Framingham Massachusetts Heart Study – a longitudinal study of heart disease among several thousand inhabitants of the town of the same name. 'Framingham', as it became known, was adapted, manipulated, and promoted to support the hypothesis that dietary cholesterol is bad for human health and should be avoided – a hypothesis eventually broadened to include saturated fats as well. The conclusions of the Framingham Study were announced with great fanfare, much of it from government agencies who also helped to promote margarine's new identity as the healthy alternative to butter and its saturated fat.

North Americans willingly adapted their diets to reflect the implications of the lipid hypothesis. Abstaining from saturated fats, and adopting aspects of the healthy diets of 'international' cuisine, didn't seem like such difficult adjustments to make if they benefited health and added years to your life. But all that heart-healthy international cuisine had to be North Americanised before we would eat it; North Americans did not embrace oil drizzled on bread, like the Italians, or Portuguese-style fish soup, or fresh sardines dripping in virgin oils, like the Spanish, or the miso tofu soup eaten in Japan. And so oil was made into hydrogenated margarine, and tofu from the orient was made into soy milk, soy hot dogs, and (of course) soy hamburgers. Pasta with oil and herbs from Italy was served in trough-size portions, hidden under copious amounts of rich sauces and topped with reconstituted Parmesan cheese product from a cardboard container. (This would surely appal the Italians, who use sauce sparingly on small servings of pasta richly laden with fresh herbs.)

In short, we didn't actually adopt the healthy habits of international cuisine; the foods produced for North Americans, while *styled* on the healthier cuisines of other cultures, were made from inferior products that were subsequently processed, packaged, artificially coloured, and marketed in forms that made them seem more familiar and acceptable. And then they were all presented in mammoth servings. In short, what started out as the promotion of a healthier 'international' diet for Americans simply resulted in the opening up of whole new realms of marketing for the processed food industry. Americans did not eliminate American cuisine from their diets and *substitute* the virgin fresh products of Ancel Keys' research. They were merely given more food choices, and subjected to a whole new set of marketing images and promises and fears, all revolving around notions of 'health'.

The result is that we can justifiably ask whether any health improvements at all have resulted from all these changes. The margarine mentality has been spread thickly over all that we eat. Saturated fat got a bad rap more than forty years ago, but its systematic elimination from our diet in favour of unsaturated fats has not done anything to ameliorate the distinctly North American health problems this change was supposed to eliminate. North Americans continue to suffer from heart attacks, cancer, arthritis, obesity and diabetes – now more than ever! The switch to unsaturated fat has not done what it was supposed to do.

It is time to re-evaluate the merits of saturated fats and reconsider returning to our dietary roots, with a diet rich in wholesome eggs, meat, dairy, whole non-refined grains, fruits, and vegetables topped with lots and lots of butter. It is my goal to demonstrate the outrageously unscientific nature of the current 'ideologies' around fats: the generic oversimplification of the categories into which fats are crowbarred, the arbitrarily restricted levels of fat consumption recommended in 'food guides', and the across-the-board vilification of saturated fats. In the pursuit of sustained good health, it is vital to incorporate all of nature's wonderful, nutritious and satisfying fats and lipids. In all of human history, no people free from the ravages of famine or plague has ever been so unhealthy, so young, as we are. Perhaps a little bit of butter could help.

Chapter 3

How The Body Uses Fats

How our ideas about fat have changed

If people were going to abandon the saturated fats they loved, and embrace a diet rich in vegetable oils, information had to be circulated in a consumer-friendly form that would convince people to spread margarine instead of butter, to eat chicken instead of red meat, and to use shortening instead of lard. I can remember the fervour with which my mother read all the health guidelines that were beginning to appear when I was a young child. In large part her motivation was simply to stay slim, as no man would want a fat woman with six children under the age of 13 – bad enough a slim woman with such a brood. And of course in the end it's easier to get rid of kids than fat on your hips, since the kids grow up and move out, but the hips just hang around, getting older and fatter.

The population back then was just getting accustomed to food guidelines, and to being bombarded with nutrition-themed information in every sort of print media, some long-established and some quite new, such as the pocket size booklets listing the calorie counts of every sort of food that were appearing at the checkouts of grocery stores. As consumers became more experienced at absorbing nutrition information, these booklets began to list the actual fat, protein and carbohydrate content of fresh and processed foods. My mother always had these handy little booklets floating around the house, and I had all the numbers and values memorised before I was 12 years old. I knew the caloric penalty of every food, but had no real understanding of nutrition until my mid-twenties.

Around this time, the nutrition-conscious consumer began to be introduced to a new set of analogies and metaphors about how their diets affected their health. This seems to be something that people are predisposed to do anyway – perhaps it's something left over from the days when our instincts and cultures actually led us to healthy foods. In any event, these analogies and metaphors circulated widely, till they eventually became accepted by consumers as descriptions of real biological processes, rather than as the over-simplifying metaphors they so often were. This is the most basic way in which we understood food. People all around the world understand food and nutrition – wisely or unwisely, depending on the time and place – according to metaphors and images from the world around them. Two things changed in the modern era: first, a new set of actors appeared, with the resources to convince us that we needed the foods they were manufacturing in their modern, hygienic, high-tech factories. And second, we began to base our metaphors and images of how fat worked on something that seemed to be rooted in real science, instead of in the folkloric notions of the past. This gave them a new kind of authority, akin to the authority of doctors and scientists and engineers.

And in the new urban mythology of nutrition, saturated fat played a central role, as a hard fat that clogs arteries and blood, because it is solid at room temperature. This probably also comes from the obvious analogy with how fat acts outside our bodies, where we can see it; if you pour liquid saturated fat from cooking down the drain without pouring hot water after it, the saturated fats will congeal and clog the drain. It's an easy step from this everyday experience to images of saturated fats doing the same in your arteries and heart and blood.

My mother always poured the bacon fat down the drain with a stream of hot water right along with it. My Grandmother, on the other hand, would never throw out the bacon fat. She would save it in that recycled jam jar and use it elsewhere. It's surely true that if you pour liquid fats down the drain they can clog things up, but this has absolutely nothing to do with how the body uses saturated fats. You are not made of pipes and drains; you are a complex system of tissue, cells, mediated hormones, blood, and electrical impulses. Your body does not clog up when you ingest saturated fats, and in any event no-one drinks pans filled with liquid fats, saturated or unsaturated. The drain analogy of saturated fat is a fragment of mythology that helped dissuade so many women from serving up butter and beef. You may *feel* like the kitchen sink some days, but in no way does your body deal with saturated fats like the drain under the sink does. Hopefully, after reading this book you'll save the bacon fat too, and stop pouring all that nutrition down the drain.

The desaturase system

Human biology has a system for dealing with all the fats we ingest – all the natural ones. I know Grandma Doolittle didn't know all the biological details about fat metabolism, but she knew that fats were inherently different, even the ones that looked the same, like lard and tallow. Grandma always used a variety of fats in that little kitchen at the top of the cellar stairs. Without knowing it, she was collaborating with the human *enzymatic desaturase system* – the system that, when necessary, breaks ingested fats down into other dietary fats according to our bodies' needs. This process helps regulate and optimise ratios of all the necessary fatty acids, and also stimulates inflammatory and anti-inflammatory reactions. The desaturase system is a critical pathway for fat metabolism, and its proper functioning depends on the availability of optimum levels and ratios of the different fats – which depends in turn on our *eating* these fats in healthy amounts and proportions.

Our desaturase enzyme system is a body rhythm that automatically adjusts to maintain the internal balance of fats available to our body, in accordance with its nutritional needs. The term 'desaturase' just means to make something unsaturated, and the '-ase' ending means that this is achieved by means of enzymes. Basically, this system functions by inserting a double bond and simultaneously removing two hydrogen atoms from the fatty acid. (You'll understand all this by the end of the book – I promise!) *Through the desaturase enzyme system, saturated fatty acids can be changed into unsaturated fatty acids!* When you eat a steak, with its triglycerides rich in saturated stearic acid, your body desaturates that fat (if it isn't all melted off during cooking) into monounsaturated oleic acid – the same fatty acid dominant in olive oil. And when you eat palm oil, the saturated fat once used in commercial frying and in so many processed foods before it was replaced with canola and vegetable oil, the desaturase enzyme system can desaturate it into stearic acid, and then again (further) into oleic acid. This is an important process, because it allows us to eat saturated fats for their many benefits, such as stability when heated, and still desaturate them if our system doesn't need as much as we've taken in.

How efficient and effective your systems of desaturation are will depend on your overall nutrition, the balance of fats in your system and diet, and your exposure to environmental or emotional stress. The desaturase system functions better in some people than others, but in general, the more healthily you eat the better this system will work. The desaturase system has evolved to help maintain human health by producing almost all the fats needed by the body, using just a few essential fats as raw material. The automatic system of double bonding upon which the system is based is catalysed by enzymes made from vitamin B6 and minerals zinc, iron and magnesium. Fresh vegetables are the best fuel for this enzymatic process, as they tend to be rich in magnesium. Other effective fuels are bran, figs, wheat germ, fish, milk, spinach, nuts, dairy, and seafood. B6 is found in leafy greens, peas, prunes, whole grains, as well as in meat, brewers yeast and molasses, while good sources of zinc include brewers yeast, nuts, dark poultry, seeds, spinach, seafood, soybeans, and whole grains. Iron is found in dried fruits of all kinds, in red meat, dark green vegetables, chickpeas and molasses. All these foods help drive the desaturase mechanism that helps metabolise our fats.

In summary; zinc, magnesium, B6 and iron are the nutrients essential to the transformation of saturated fatty acids into unsaturated fatty acids. Your body is always juggling the available raw materials – the fats in your diet – to make the best fuel available. But the desaturation pathway can be inhibited; excessive blood cholesterol can slow the conversion of all fats, and trans fatty acids, high levels of sugar or alcohol or low levels of zinc, magnesium, B6 or iron will bog the system down. The human desaturase system is a marvellous endogenous balancing tool, but it is often placed under a tremendous burden. We will discuss, in the chapter on essential fatty acids, one of the most significant aspects of this burden: the conversion of omega 3 and 6 fatty acids and the effect our modern diet has on this process.

The key ingredients that slow down fatty acid desaturation and fatty acid conversion

- Trans fatty acids from hydrogenation: Trans fatty acids are found in margarine, shortening, and hydrogenated spreads like peanut butter and Nutella.
- *Excess* animal trans fats: These are higher in commercial beef than in beef from grass fed cattle.
- Artificially polyunsaturated fats found in margarine, shortenings, cookies, pastries, spreads such as peanut butter, crackers and breads.
- Excess vegetable oil, such as vegetable oil blends, corn oil, safflower oil, canola oil. In excess, it dominates the desaturase system and hogs enzymes also needed by other pathways.
- Low calorie diets, resulting in insufficient micro-nutrients to drive the system.
- Excess cholesterol, which can come from excess sugars and starch as well as from fats.
- Excess alcohol
- Excess saturated fat intake (meat or dairy eaten in excess will tax the enzymes available to desaturate the saturated fats.
- Excess calories

The body's systems of desaturation function best when supplied with a little bit of all the fats, but not with too much of any one of them, or with too many calories overall.

Fatty Acid Desaturation Pathways

Omega 3 rich fats are found in flaxseed, hemp, rapeseed, unrefined soybean, dark green leafy vegetables and walnuts. These omega 3 fats are derived from food sources and cannot be made in the body. They encounter the delta 9 desaturase enzyme in their first conversion towards longer chain super unsaturated fatty acids.

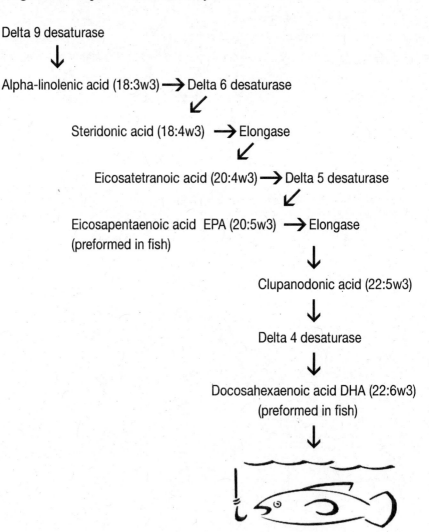

Delta 9 desaturase

↓

Alpha-linolenic acid (18:3w3) → Delta 6 desaturase

↙

        Steridonic acid (18:4w3) → Elongase

↙

            Eicosatetranoic acid (20:4w3) → Delta 5 desaturase

↙

      Eicosapentaenoic acid EPA (20:5w3) → Elongase
(preformed in fish)

↓

          Clupanodonic acid (22:5w3)

↓

          Delta 4 desaturase

↓

       Docosahexaenoic acid DHA (22:6w3)
(preformed in fish)

↓

Omega 6 rich fats are found at 20% or more concentration in mixed vegetable oils, canola oil, corn oil, cottonseed oil, sesame oil, soybean oil, sunflower oil, safflower oil, grape seed oil, peanut oil and walnut oil. The omega 6 rich fats are derived from foods and cannot be made in our bodies. They encounter the delta 9 desaturase enzyme in their first conversion towards super unsaturated fatty acids.

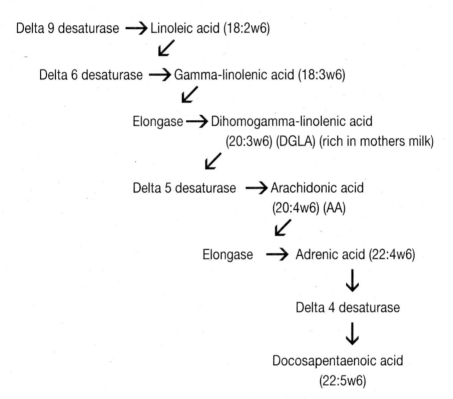

Delta 9 desaturase ⟶ Linoleic acid (18:2w6)

Delta 6 desaturase ⟶ Gamma-linolenic acid (18:3w6)

Elongase ⟶ Dihomogamma-linolenic acid
(20:3w6) (DGLA) (rich in mothers milk)

Delta 5 desaturase ⟶ Arachidonic acid
(20:4w6) (AA)

Elongase ⟶ Adrenic acid (22:4w6)

Delta 4 desaturase

Docosapentaenoic acid
(22:5w6)

Omega 9 fatty acids in concentrations greater than 22% are found in almonds, beef tallow, butterfat, human butterfat, canola oil, cocoa butter, cod liver oil (only 22%), corn oil, flaxseed oil (only 21%), lard, olive oil, palm oil, palm olein, palm kernel, peanut oil, sesame oil, soybean oil and walnut oil. Unlike the omega 3 and 6 fatty acids, omega 9 fatty acids can be manufactured within the body. Acetate fragments accumulate from excess carbohydrate, protein or fat intake. These fragments combine to form myristic fatty acid, a 14 carbon chain fat. From there they can proceed to form saturated fatty acids palmitic or stearic acid. Stearic acid encounters the delta 9 desaturase enzyme as the first step towards desaturation.

Stearic acid (18:0) (Stearic acid is the fat rich in red meats)

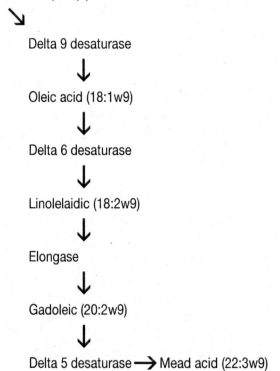

Delta 9 desaturase

↓

Oleic acid (18:1w9)

↓

Delta 6 desaturase

↓

Linolelaidic (18:2w9)

↓

Elongase

↓

Gadoleic (20:2w9)

↓

Delta 5 desaturase ⟶ Mead acid (22:3w9)

Omega 7 fatty acids come from food sources of palm oil family and coconut as well as being manufactured within the body from excess acetate fragments. Palmitic acid is a 16 carbon saturated fatty acid that encounters delta 9 desaturase enzyme as the first step towards omega 7 desaturation.

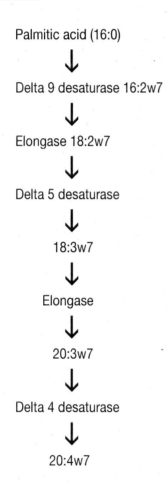

Palmitic acid (16:0)

↓

Delta 9 desaturase 16:2w7

↓

Elongase 18:2w7

↓

Delta 5 desaturase

↓

18:3w7

↓

Elongase

↓

20:3w7

↓

Delta 4 desaturase

↓

20:4w7

Cell membranes are made of fat and our bodies are made up of cells

Cells are progressively organized into tissues, and tissues into organs. Organs co-ordinate to function as systems, and together these systems make up the whole human body. So the human body is entirely made of living cells that are organized to sustain life. All the organs, including the brain, heart, lungs, liver, kidney, pancreas, skin, spleen and stomach, and all the systems that function along with these organs; muscles, tendons, ligaments, intestines, bladder, blood, and cartilage... all of these are made up of cells! And fats play a crucial role in maintaining the health and integrity of every one of these cells; fats are the main constituents of the membrane called the *lipid bilayer* that surrounds all cells. The lipid bilayer is typically two layers deep (hence the name) and made of special fats called phospholipids, as well as cholesterol, protein and minute portions of carbohydrates. Our bodies depend on the nutrients that constitute and maintain the lipid bilayer. These fatty cell membranes are a critical defence mechanism for all cells; they are the gatekeepers that control the ebb and flow of nutrients and of non-nutrient particles. So we can say that the health of cell membranes is crucial to the health of the entire body, which is therefore dependent on a steady supply of quality fats, along with the co-nutrients that metabolise these fats.

The cell membranes of different organs and systems are made up of different concentrations of lipids. How much cholesterol a cell membrane contains depends on how much unsaturated fat is built into the cell's phospholipids. Highly unsaturated cell membranes, built from unsaturated dietary fat, will gradually accumulate cholesterol, which will be integrated into the membrane to give it a little more stiffness and integrity. This is the major reason why diets high in polyunsaturated fat are successful at reducing blood cholesterol; the cells integrate the unsaturated fat, and cholesterol is removed from the circulating blood to strengthen the cellular membranes.

A cell is in many ways an entity unto itself. The organelles housed within each cell have specific roles to keep the cells healthy and functioning, and are also surrounded by their own lipid membranes. There are components called mitochondria that allow the cell to 'breathe' by producing chemical energy. The lysosomes constitute the digestive system of the cell, while endoplasmic reticula help the cell form new membranes and manufacture products for secretion. The Golgi complex distributes new synthesized proteins, and peroxisomes detoxify individual cells. The DNA is found in the nucleus of the cell and houses the genetic information needed for replication. To function efficiently and to maintain homeostasis (a relatively stable internal environment) a cell and all its compartments must be contained within a healthy membrane wall – a lipid bilayer made of just the right proportions of fats, cholesterol, proteins and phospholipids.

Phospholipids

There are many different phospholipids. Different cell membranes have different amounts and proportions of fat, but most of these fats are phospholipids. Coupled with cholesterol, the phospholipids provide the necessary integrity for all cell walls, ensuring that the membrane is neither too soft nor too stiff. A phospholipid is made up of two fatty acids, largely derived from the food we eat, one vitamin-like phosphorous-rich molecule, and a simple organic molecule such as inositol, choline, ethanolamine or serine. These last two are also common vitamin supplements promoted for cognitive enhancement.

The most common phospholipids are: *phosphatidylcholine* (lecithin is its more common name), *phosphatidylethanolamine, phosphatidylserine* and *phosphatidylinositol.* An important thing to understand about these phospholipids is that the fatty acids within a particular type of phospholipid will be different in different tissues. Thus the phosphatidylcholine of the brain may be composed of different fatty acids than the phosphatidylcholine of the lungs. This clearly demonstrates the importance of fat variety in our diet, since all the different phospholipids will use different fatty acids within their structure. The arbitrary elimination of entire categories of fat from one's diet could be a game of Russian roulette.

For example, the most common phospholipid within the brain is phosphatidylcholine. The two dominant fatty acids in the phosphatidylcholine within the brain are palmitic acid and oleic acid. Palmitic acid is a major component of palm oil, which has been a forbidden saturated fat throughout the last 25 years of nutrition recommendations, while oleic acid is derived from olive oil and is the monounsaturated fat that is so widely promoted for heart health. However *both* these fatty acids are critical to the healthy functioning of the brain's dominant phospholipid. Instead of oleic and palmitic acids, the phosphatidylcholine of the lungs is ideally made up of choline (a vitamin-like molecule) and two saturated palmitic fatty acids, again made from the palm oil that is regarded in solely negative terms in current received wisdom. The phosphatidylserine of the brain is made up of stearic acid, a saturated fatty acid found predominately in red meats, and oleic acid, the monounsaturated fatty acid found in olive oil. In the phosphatidylcholine of red blood cells, on the other hand, the fatty acids are palmitic and linoleic from omega 6 rich fats.

The principles underlying the functions of cell membranes and their phospholipids are fundamental to understanding the arguments presented in this book. Phospholipids are clearly one of the major building blocks of the human body, and their maintenance requires a significant supply of saturated fats. More than 50% of the body's phospholipids are constructed of saturated fatty acids. And remember; these saturated fatty acids are derived from the food we eat. Optimum cell membrane flexibility and permeability are dependent on adequate supplies of the fatty acids of phospholipids and cholesterol molecules, which enable communication within the cell, and between the cell and its environment, as well as regulating cell life. Too much polyunsaturated fat, or not enough saturated fat, will result in imbalanced cell membranes with inefficient nutrient flow and communication. In other words, your cells will be unhealthy, inefficient, and at risk of degeneration and death. There is a critical need for saturated fats, and all natural lipids, in human nutrition; but this fact has been negated, obscured and forgotten in all the recommendations to 'avoid saturated fats'. These have misled people into believing there are no direct health benefits from saturated fat when in fact, as we can see from the description of phospholipids, saturated fat is an *essential life force*.

The need for minerals and vitamins to fuel the desaturation process is just one example of the great diversity of nutrients needed by the human body if it is to maintain optimal health. The body's various systems will slow down or work inefficiently with too few calories, while foods dense in nutrients will drive the metabolism. Low calorie diets are generally low in *micronutrients* such as iron, zinc, B6, and magnesium, all needed to drive many aspects of fat metabolism. If you adhere to a low calorie, low fat diet on a regular basis, you'll likely be assimilating insufficient vitamin and mineral micronutrients to fuel the body's calorie burning system, which will actually slow down. And if calorie restriction is habitual, the low nutrient intake that goes with it is believed to cause the metabolism to slow down *permanently*. So it is that the long-chain saturated fats of beef, pork, and dairy products, when they form part of a wholesome diet, will enrich and benefit overall health and contribute to a faster metabolism. Saturated fat from animal sources also provides iron, B12, zinc, and carnitine, all of which are essential for optimal health and the metabolism of fat itself.

How much fat should you eat? Opinions vary on this issue, and if you compare sources within the nutritional literature, you'll find they offer divergent advice about our need for fat, and very different recommendations about how much fat we should eat. The minimum human fat requirement is approximately 1½ tablespoons per 100 pounds of lean body mass. (Lean body mass is your body weight without fat). This 1½ tablespoons would include the oils naturally present in our food, not just oil added to foods or taken as supplements. An adult who's neither overweight nor underweight will have an average of about 22% body fat – men a little less, women a little more. So if you're relatively healthy, and an average weight for your height, just subtract 22% of your total body weight to get your lean body mass; a 125 pound woman should consume a minimum of (125 - 22% = 96 lbs) about 1½ tablespoons, and a 180 pound man a minimum of (180 – 20% = 144) just over two. Here's a more user-friendly method; eat foods rich in quality fat two or three times a day. This will get you to your quota and not put you over. And minimise the amount of fat you use for cooking; it should make up the smallest proportion of the fat that you eat, since cooked fat is generally less good for you than raw fat.

Fat is our friend. The human body has incredibly sophisticated methods of dealing with all the *natural* fats we consume, as long as we consume them in sensible amounts. In fact, variety is exactly what we need when it comes to fat consumption. The chapters that follow will hopefully make this clear, by showing how fats are constructed, and how different fats serve a host of different purposes in our bodies.

CHAPTER 4
THE NITTY GRITTY BIOCHEMISTRY OF ALL FATS

Definitions

There are four terms used in this book that mean slightly different things, and perhaps it is a good idea to make the differences between them clear before we get any further in the biochemistry. The terms are fat, lipid, oil and fatty acid. Fat and lipid do actually mean pretty much the same, though lipid is a more technical term, and includes things that are not, strictly speaking, fats; they are general terms to describe all the substances that are going to be discussed in this chapter. An oil is simply a fat that's liquid at room temperature. Finally, fat and oil are terms usually used to describe the substances we find in our kitchen or neighbourhood store –'olive oil', or 'chicken fat'. But these are actually made up of different substances, different fat molecules, and these distinct molecules, each of which has its own structure and its own functions in the human body, are 'fatty acids'. They're the red and blue and green Smarties in the box of plain old Smarties.

Triglycerides

While the structure of any one of the many fats in our diet is distinct from all the others, 95 percent of them are *triglycerides*. The triglycerides, along with the phospholipids that make up the cell membranes, are the fats that we will be most concerned with in this book. The term "tri-glyceride" describes the physical composition of these fats. '*Tri-*' refers to the three fatty acids swimming off the end of the *glycerol* molecule; glycerol is a three-carbon molecule that makes up the backbone of

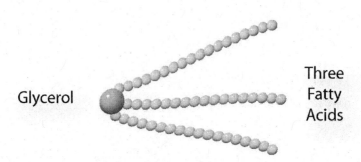

Glycerol

Three Fatty Acids

Tryiglyceride, showing the glycerol base and the three fatty acid chains.

the triglyceride, and the fatty acids anchor onto this. They look like three caterpillars hanging from a short twig.

The *length* of these three fatty acids, and the number and concentration of hydrogen molecules attached to them, will determine the function of a triglyceride within the body, as well as how it is named and categorized. Triglycerides are space-saving molecules; they are very densely structured compared to carbohydrates and protein, and so make great storage fuel for the body. They transport the fat-soluble vitamins A, D, E, and K, and they are used in the making of phospholipids and spingolipids (which constitute the membranes of nerve tissue). If triglycerides are broken down through oxidation before we consume them, the oil quality deteriorates, producing low-molecular-weight compounds that give oil a distinct and unpleasant odour and flavour. In addition, the oxidized oil produces toxic compounds and destroys essential fatty acids that yield building blocks for cholesterol synthesis. Too much of any type of triglyceride, saturated or unsaturated, can affect cholesterol levels. This is an important aspect of the relationship between cholesterol, unsaturated fats, and high blood cholesterol, but one that is virtually ignored in the health promotion of unsaturated fats.

Fatty acids (the caterpillars) attach to the glycerol molecule twig in a variety of patterns. There are three positions to which fatty acids can attach themselves; position 1 is at the top of the glycerol molecule, position 2 in the middle, and position 3 at the bottom. The fatty acids' order on the glycerol will affect how the molecule is chosen for digestion and metabolism. The greater the variety of fats in the diet, the greater the diversity of fatty acid arrays on the triglycerides available for use within the body. This is further support for the principle of not eating predominately one type of fat while avoiding others.

Just what is a saturated fat?

When a fatty acid carbon chain is filled to capacity with hydrogen atoms it is defined as *saturated*. This means that the molecule of fat cannot accept another hydrogen atom and is 'saturated' with hydrogen; the carbon chain cannot host any more hydrogen. Remember how we imagined every fatty acid chain as a caterpillar dangling from a twig. Now if we were to start putting tiny little hydrogen shoes on a caterpillar's feet until there was no room for any more, this caterpillar/fatty acid chain would be saturated. Predominantly saturated fats have higher melting temperatures than other fats, and consequently they are more resistant to burning or denaturing. (Think of saturated fats having greater stability because all those hydrogen shoes on the fatty acid caterpillar keep the creature still and not so active.) To be defined as saturated, a fat has to have a minimum of 10% of its constituent fat molecules in a saturated form. At this point it will be hard at room temperature, not liquid like oils. So if 10% of the fatty acid caterpillars have *all* their hydrogen shoes on, the fat will behave as saturated. For the most part, it's correct to assume that hard fats are saturated fats and vice versa. However, some shorter chain saturated fats, like coconut oil, can be liquid at room temperature. Clearly we have to stop using general rules of thumb to categorise fats and oils, and try to understand the complexities of all fats in a bit more depth.

Unsaturated oils do not have hydrogen atoms on every carbon. Their caterpillars only wear hydrogen shoes on every third set of feet, so they are not heavy with shoes, or tightly packed together. Every third set of legs has a double bond that allows them to be light – to bend and twist and move around easily, because there is room for the fatty acid to do so. And so unsaturated oils spread out and drip. Oils are just fats, or '*lipids*' that are liquid at room temperature. Some of the most common unsaturated fats and oils in our diets are olive, safflower, sunflower, soybean, corn, canola and grape seed oils, and last but not least... lard. Lard, despite all the promotion that it is a saturated fat, is mostly unsaturated.

Olive and grape seed oils are different from the others in that they're missing just one pair of shoes and have only one double bond.

Nature's Critical Ratio

There is an endogenous balancing system (one taking place within our bodies) that nutrition science terms the 'critical ratio'. This critical ratio is the optimum balance between a particular pair of constituent elements found in both saturated and unsaturated fatty acids. This balance ensures that an animal's desaturase enzyme systems can metabolise all fats efficiently, and so reap the greatest health benefits from each one. The unsaturated portion of animal fat needs to contain a minimum ratio of 1 part linoleic or 'omega 6' fatty acid to 19 parts oleic or 'omega 9' fatty acid to avoid an unbalanced competition for the enzymes that break down the fats. If the ratio of omega 6 to omega 9 dips below this level, the health benefits of linoleic acid (omega 6, or O6) are lost, as the enzymes that metabolise it are monopolised by the demands of the oleic acid (O9). This results in the fatty acids in meat remaining unchanged at the end of metabolising, minimizing their nutritional value. In pigs, oleic acid constitutes about 87% of unsaturated fats and linoleic acid about 12.3%. This makes pork fats relatively healthy, as the ratio between the O9 and O6 is well above 5%. Our body's enzyme system would be able to produce enough enzymes to efficiently metabolise and utilize both the linoleic acid *and* the omega 9, and not just store either as adipose tissue (stored fat) – which is what occurs when a diet contains insufficient variety or unbalanced ratios of fat.

Domesticated, corn-fed cattle do not fare as well as pork. They miss the critical ratio by a 'small rump roast'. Their unsaturated fats contain roughly 97% oleic acid to only 2.55% linoleic acid. This means their linoleic fatty acid will not be as *bioavailable,* since in such small proportions it will not be provided with the enzymes it needs to offer its health benefits to the body.

But animal feed has a great influence on the fat quality and ratios of an animal; grass-fed cattle have higher concentrations of conjugated linoleic acid, and different fat ratios than grain-fed cattle. Wild animals that forage have very different fatty acid profiles than domesticated animals; they are much more varied. And a greater variety of fatty acids within meats results in less competition for the enzymes needed to break down the fats. This ensures that the endogenous response to the fats will also be varied, allowing the body to carry out a wider range of processes on these fats, and put them to a greater and more balanced range of uses. Contrary to current guidelines and dogma, the saturated fats in red meat are healthful. There are many uses for these fats. And preparing meat in a variety of ways, buying meat from different suppliers (in order to get meat raised under different feeding regimes), eating wild game when it is available, and eating organic are all practical ways to recreate the fatty acid variety found in meat produced before the age of industrial, monoculture farming.

Saturated Fats: Summary of Health Benefits

- Enhances the immune system
- Necessary for healthy bones, used for calcium assimilation
- Provides energy by short and medium chain fatty acids
- Enhances structural integrity of cells
- Its stability allows for longer shelf life
- Improves anti-oxidant status
- Stable for high-heat cooking and manufacturing
- 18c stearic has neutral cholesterol affect
- 16c and 18c fatty acids are preferred fuels for the heart
- Transports fat-soluble vitamins
- Short chain saturates are not stored in adipose tissue
- Anti-microbial properties maintain a healthy gut
- Eliminate the need for hydrogenated products

CHAPTER 5
SATURATED FATTY ACIDS / SAFA

"…As the science has advanced, we know more and more that the way we used to simply group all fats into one basket and equate them isn't the way the biology works" [1] (My Grandma Doolittle knew that!)

Science marches on:

For over four decades saturated fats have been condemned for their deleterious "artery clogging" effects. Many authoritative medical sources have advised decreasing the consumption of all saturated fats, because of their presumed effects on blood cholesterol levels and heart disease. However, it is now an established scientific fact that many saturated fats have beneficial biological effects – that they are in fact essential for optimal health. Many medium chain fats support our immune system, help the body absorb minerals, and are an important source of fuel, especially for infants, athletes and individuals with impaired fat assimilation. Studies that deal with specific fatty acids and their effect, or non-effect, on serum cholesterol levels have shown that only one commonly-consumed fat, *myristic acid,* increases the level of cholesterol in the blood, while the rest have no effect at all on blood lipid profiles.

All saturated fats are not equal! Uncritical acceptance of the catch-all term 'saturated fat', and the assumption that it describes a set of substances that are in practical terms the same, has led public food policy and consumers a long long way down the wrong path. Saturated fat is in fact a varied and complicated collection of substances, and should never be ascribed a single set of qualities and effects. Nutrition policies that advocate for puritanical reductions in all dietary saturated fats have lead North Americans steadily towards a state of totally imbalanced fat consumption.

And the practise of simply assuming that animal fats are saturated is also misleading and wrong; if we look at their constituent fats, and *their* fatty acid profiles, we can see that most animal fats are more unsaturated than saturated. This fact, coupled with a dramatically increased consumption of polyunsaturated fat, means that most people have diets *too low* in saturated fats. Saturated fat is healthful and essential; it cannot be marginalized and vilified any longer.

Some misunderstood aspects of saturated fatty acids

1) Fats and oils do not contain triglyceride molecules with only one type of fatty acid. Saturated fats have a combination of saturated and unsaturated fatty acid chains. They are categorized as saturated fats if 10% or more of their triglycerides are saturated.
2) Saturated fats can contain short or long-chain fatty acids, *and chain length has more affect on a fat's healthfulness than its saturation point does.* This is one of the most critical and misunderstood aspects of saturated fats.
3) Not all saturated fats are digested and assimilated in the same way. Therefore all fats affect blood lipid profiles differently.
4) All triglycerides have fatty acids attached to a glycerol backbone. The order of the fatty acids on the backbone plays an important role in the fat's physiological effects. This is true for saturated fats as well.
5) Saturated fats contain essential nutrients other than fatty acids. Palm oil, for example, is the *richest* source of the anti-oxidant beta carotene and a rich source of Vitamin E.
6) Our vital organs, including our heart and lungs, depend on a source of saturated fatty acids for fuel.

Sources of saturated fatty acids

There are 13 known natural saturated fatty acids. They vary in chain length from 4 to 24 carbons, and because they are saturated with hydrogen there are no double bonds. The saturated fat in the foods we commonly eat contain eight of these saturated fatty acids; the five others are not present in significant amounts in our diets. The *natural* saturated fats that we consume (as opposed to the fats found in shortening and margarine, artificially saturated by hydrogenation) and their fatty acid profiles are as follows:

- *Lard*, rendered from pork fat. 40% saturated; 48% monounsaturated; 12% polyunsaturated (40% of the caterpillar fatty acids have all of their hydrogen shoes on; 48% of the caterpillars forgot one pair of shoes; 12% of caterpillars put shoes on in pairs of three, missing several sets of feet). Of the saturated fat in lard, 2% is 14-carbon myristic acid, (medium chain fatty acid), 23-26% the 16-carbon palmitic acid, 14% is 18-carbon stearic acid.
- *Tallow*, from beef fat. 49% saturated; 49% monounsaturated; 4% polyunsaturated. Tallow's saturated fat is 3% is 14 carbon myristic, 24% is 16-carbon palmitic, 19% is 18-carbon stearic.
- *Palm Oil*, from the flesh of the palm plant. 50% saturated; 40% unsaturated; 10% polyunsaturated. 1% is 14-carbon myristic, 45% 16-carbon palmitic, 4% 18-carbon stearic.
- *Butter*, from the milk of cows. 55% saturated; 23 % monounsaturated; 3% polyunsaturated. 4% of butter's saturated fat is 4-carbon butyric, 3 % is 10-carbon capric, 3% 12-carbon lauric, 11% is 14-carbon myristic, 27% is 16-carbon palmitic, and 12% is 18-carbon stearic.
- *Cocoa Butter*, from the cocoa bean, used predominantly in candy. 61% saturated; 34% unsaturated; 3% polyunsaturated. Of the saturated cocoa butter, 25% is 16-carbon palmitic acid, 38% is 18-carbon stearic acid.
- *Palm Kernel Oil*, from the nut of the palm plant. 78% saturated; 15% monounsaturated; 2% polyunsaturated. In palm kernel oil, 4% of saturated fat is 8-carbon caprylic, 4% is 10-carbon capric, 48% is 12-carbon lauric acid, 16% is 14-carbon myristic, 8% is 16-carbon palmitic, 3% is 18-carbon stearic acid.
- *Coconut Oil*, from coconuts. 92% saturated; 6% monounsaturated; 2% polyunsaturated. Of the saturated fats in coconut oil, 49% is the 12-carbon lauric acid, 8% 8-carbon caprylic acid, 7% 10-carbon

capric acid, 18% 14-carbon myristic acid, 9% 16-carbon palmitic acid, 3% is 18-carbon stearic acid.

It should be clear from the above list that there are important differences between all of the saturated fats. They contain different fatty acids, in different proportions, and they all affect physiological functions in different ways.

Short Chain Saturated Fatty Acids

In the steady bombardment of nutrition information and advice unleashed on the public, no distinction is made between the different saturated fats on the basis of their chain lengths. By lumping all saturated fats together into a single undifferentiated category, food 'authorities' ignore all the health benefits that short chain saturated fats offer. One of the greatest distortions of the 'they're all the same' school of thought is that short chain fats have been found 'guilty by association' in research results that condemn *all* saturated fats as fattening, cholesterolemic and predisposing to heart disease. Short chain saturated fatty acids are not found in adipose tissue, so the fat deposits on your body contain no butter; it's not a butter bum! Short chain saturated fatty acids from dairy are still categorized simply as saturated fats, and everyone knows them as such. Public health policy directives call for saturated fat be limited to 10% of our total fat intake, regardless of fatty acid chain length. This recommendation is generally followed by examples of foods to avoid and their recommended substitutes – such as low fat dairy products in place of their natural full fat alternatives.

So foods with a higher concentration of short chain fats are not recognized as any different from foods containing other saturated fats. Butyric (4-carbon), caproic (6-carbon), caprylic (8-carbon), and capric (10-carbon) are the short chain fatty acids found in butter and buttermilk, and in goat products such as goat's milk yogurt, goat cheese, and of course goat's milk itself. (Caproic, capric and caprylic come from the Latin word for goat, as in 'Capricorn'.) Milk fat is rich in both short chain (4-10 carbon) and medium chain (10-16 carbon) saturated fats. Remember that these are all saturated fatty acids that have all their carbon molecules filled (saturated) with hydrogen atoms (the caterpillar has all his shoes on). But these are *short chains*, so there are very few carbons needing to be cleaved off and metabolised.

Medium chain saturated fatty acids

'Medium chain fatty acids' are generally defined as fatty acids between 12 and 15 carbons in length, though some sources use the term for chains 10 to 14 carbons long. The most important medium-chain fatty acids are found in coconut oil, palm kernel oil, and butterfat – foods we have systematically removed from our food supply. Lauric acid is the most abundant medium chain fatty acid. It is 12 carbons long, and predominant (47%) in coconut fat. Myristic acid is a 14-carbon fatty acid. It is relatively rare in our natural food supply, but coconut oil has 18%, palm kernel oil 16%, cod liver oil, butterfat goat and cow all less than 11%, palm olein, palm oil, lard, cottonseed oil all less than 2%,.

Medium chain fatty acids can be manufactured by means of a chemical process that involves collecting all the medium chain fatty acids from triglycerides which have a mix of fatty acid chain lengths and then combining them into new triglycerides with only medium chain fatty acids attached to the glycerol. This means that all the caterpillars (fatty acids) would be the same length and – oh my god – they are all wearing the same style of shoes on *all* their feet. (They *must* be male caterpillars) Medium chain fatty acids are used therapeutically by individuals who cannot digest fat because, for example, they produce insufficient lipase or bile salt. Malabsorption of fat is generally due to damage to the mucosal surfaces of the small intestine, or congenital failure to produce the apoproteins that help package fat for digestion. Impaired fat absorption could cause deficiencies in fat-soluable vitamins A,D,E, and K and essential fatty acids. But the medium-chain fats are usually absorbed without problems, even by those with health issues. Medium chain fats are now being added to infant formula. They are also a popular sports supplement because they provide quick, easily digestible energy without increasing levels of the hormone insulin, as sugar does. The medium-chain fatty acids have strong anti-microbial properties (perhaps this is why they are so abundant in dairy products) they do not contribute to plasma lipoproteins (the assemblies that carry fats and cholesterol in the blood-stream) and therefore have no 'cholesterol-raising' activity, and best of all (!) they are not deposited in adipose tissue.

The Long-Chain Saturated Fatty Acids

Long-chain saturated fatty acids are 16 to 24 carbons in length. Most of the long chain saturated fatty acids in our diet are either 16 carbon palmitic acid, derived from palm oil, or 18 carbon stearic acid from beef and pork. Fatty acids longer than 18 carbons are found in very low concentrations, and only in a few foods such as peanuts and cocoa. Good sources of 16:0 and 18:0 fatty acids are red meat, lard, butter, palm oil and cottonseed oil; they are present in much lower concentrations in all other fats and oils.

Humans and other animals make their own palmitic and stearic acid out of excess carbohydrates and protein. That is how important these two saturated fats are to our physiological well-being. They can be changed in turn into both 16 and 18 carbon *monounsaturated* fatty acids to ensure all physiological needs are met. It is not until someone eats beyond their caloric needs that these essential saturated fatty acids could possibly affect blood lipid profiles, including cholesterol levels, in a negative way. In this, they are no different from any other fats we eat. In fact, much of the current research on the 18-carbon stearic acid seems to show that it has a neutral to benign effect on low density cholesterol levels. Stearic acid is only found in animal foods, and is not rendered for cooking and processing.

Palm oil has been a valued part of the human diet in many parts of the world for more than 5000 years. Unrefined palm oil is rich in the essential vitamin E, along with the anti-oxident carotenoids, tocopherols and tocotrienols. These minor non-saponifiable (can't be broken down into alcohol and salts) compounds in palm oil have been proven to be strong inhibitors of HMG-CoA reductase, the enzyme that starts the rate-limiting step in cholesterol synthesis. As such, they do the same thing as Lipitor, the most widely prescribed medication for high cholesterol. Palm oil contains 18 parts per million of cholesterol – the same as many vegetable oils.

Saturated fatty acid combinations

It's important to understand that a fat defined as 'saturated' will really only be partly saturated. Saturated fats are classified as such because a certain minimum proportion of their weight is in saturated form. The composition of the individual triglyceride molecules may vary; some will be all unsaturated with one double bond, others a combination of monounsaturates and saturates, and still others will contain polyunsaturated fatty acids. Although the composition of the individual molecules may vary, the relative proportion of fatty acids remains constant. It is very rare to encounter triglycerides with only palmitic and stearic acids, though of course the classification system used today obscures this fact. Saturated fats vary in length, order and degree of saturation, and all of these variations affect their use and how they are metabolised. A saturated fat can have different fatty acid combinations, and these will affect how it is metabolised, stored and utilized, as well as how it *aggregates*, if it aggregates at all. (The aggregation of fats, which means pretty much what it sounds like, is thought to contribute to heart disease.) When all the saturated fats were grouped into one catch-all category, the vital information about their differences, and the nutritional significance of these differences, was essentially lost. Saturated fat variation is not confusing or difficult to understand; but one does need to begin by shedding the notion that all saturated fats are the same, because as far as our health is concerned there is nothing identical about them at all.

Stability of saturated fats

Stability is a critical characteristic of fats and oils that is generally ignored in the promotion of unsaturated oils in place of saturated fat. Stability refers to how much heat, light and processing the fat can tolerate before it starts to *oxidise* and cause free radical damage to the cells of those who eat it. Oxidation involves the breaking down of the fat molecules, and we take 'antioxidants' to help prevent it happening in excess. A fat's stability is enhanced by a higher degree of saturation. Saturated fats are more stable, and cause less free radical damage than unsaturated fats when cooked, heated, processed, and metabolised. They are slower to react with other chemicals, like enzymes, which break food down into smaller usable parts, and because of this saturated fats take longer to digest. Saturated fats tend to aggregate or clump together even in the blood. Or rather: saturated fats got their "bad fat" reputation because *some of them* aggregate in the blood and, it was thought, do not react within the body because they are so stable. Upon closer examination it becomes clear that saturated fats *do* react within the body, and that the different saturated fats do so in very different ways.

Short Chain Fatty Acid Digestion

Short and medium chain fatty acids metabolise quickly, compared to their long chain cousins, because there aren't so many little boots to untie and take off. These fatty acids' 4:0-12:0 carbons can be digested without bile, (the salt that is defused from the gall bladder and that emulsifies fat during digestion) much like any carbohydrate. For the most part, short chain saturated fats use the same metabolic pathway as carbohydrates; they go through the hepatic portal system directly to the liver to be used for energy, and for other functions of fat. Even though they are saturated fats they metabolise quickly and easily, with minimum need for digestion and emulsion, and they can't be repackaged into parts of a cholesterol bundle. Basically, the short chain fats of butter, coconut, palm kernel, and goat milk have no effect at all on blood cholesterol!

It has long been recognized that the shorter the chain length of a fatty acid and the lower its molecular mass, the lower its gross energy per gram. This means that even though short chain fats are still fats, they actually contain fewer calories than longer chain fats. Because the shorter chain metabolizes very quickly and is chemically more akin to carbohydrates than long chain saturated fatty acids, the available energy of short chain fats has to be less than that of longer chain fats. The caterpillar shoes are gobbled up by the body faster than the shoes on long chain caterpillars. The 3-carbon glycerol backbone of a short chain fat has a lower calorie value than the attached fatty acids. Essentially this carbon backbone metabolises as a carbohydrate, being assimilated directly into the blood just like honey or other sugars. As the fatty acid chains get shorter (as in butter, whose profile contains four-carbon chains) this backbone makes up a greater proportion of the total caloric value. Short chain fats tend to have a caloric value of only five calories per gram, in contrast to their longer-chain cousins, which do indeed contain the nine calories per gram we've learned to fear.

It is important to understand that I am constructing an argument against the current dogma that has blacklisted all saturated fats. Some very arbitrary dietary commandments have been put forth concerning our intake of saturated fats – without any acknowledgement of the complex and diverse biochemistry that exists within every category of fats. When we indiscriminately restrict *all* saturated fats in our diet, we lose all the benefits of these fats as well.

Longer Chain Fatty Acid Digestion

The longer chain fats, from 14:0–20:0 carbons, will digest after they have been emulsified with bile salts that come from the gall bladder. Then lipase enzymes can break down the fats in the small intestine into three substances: these are *monoglycerides* (glycerol molecules with only one fatty acid chain), *free fatty acids* (fatty acids not anchored to a glycerol molecule), and *glycerol molecules* (the 3-carbon backbones that anchor the fatty acids). From the intestine they are transported to the lymphatic system and repackaged into carrier molecules called chylomicrons. The chylomicrons carry their packages of fats to tissues, and to the liver – where they are broken down again, this time into ATP molecules of energy by *beta*-oxidation or *omega*-oxidation. The different oxidative pathways refer to which end of the fatty acid digestion starts at. It's pretty much the end of the road for fats at this point; if they aren't used for energy at this stage they will be stored in the adipose tissue on your belly or butt (or the back of your arms, or your chin...)

The longer-chain saturated fats, in which beef, lamb, tallow and suet are so rich, are slower to metabolise because they don't break apart as easily as short chain saturated fatty acids such as the butyric acid of butter, the lauric acid in coconut, or the polyunsaturated fatty acids in flaxseed oil. For most people the slower breakdown of long chain saturated fats results in a strong sense of satiety, because these fats linger in the gut, allowing for the gradual release of energy. Liver and fat cells will not synthesize fat for energy while this digestion process goes on. This slower digestion is part of the reason why people tend to eat less overall when their diet is rich in saturated fats. Saturated fats lingering in the gut will stimulate other enzymes of digestion and satiety, mainly Cholecystokinin and leptin. Leptin is the hormone that communicates to your brain that you are indeed satisfied and well fed, and that you can stop eating. Cholecystokinin is a digestive enzyme that lines the walls of our small intestine, and recent research has shown that it is stimulated by an adequate intake of saturated fats. It also tells other digestive enzymes that you are well fed, and that their stimulating affect is not needed. So even if you were to smell cinnamon buns baking in the oven, and cinnamon buns were your favourite thing in the world, your body wouldn't release digestive enzymes or stimulate your appetite. You're stuffed with saturated fat and your brain knows it.

Without all this intercellular communication and brain notification it is hard to know if your body has had enough to eat. Low fat diets, and low saturated fat diets, can leave us feeling hungry and unsatisfied – a sensation any dieter knows all too well. This can, and of course usually does, lead to further eating of low-nutrient foods (like warm cinnamon buns with drippy white icing). We will only experience real satiety when all essential nutrient needs are met, including those for saturated fat.

Saturated fatty acids can be digested and assimilated in a variety of ways, and will affect health in different ways as a result; most foods containing saturated fats will provide the body with a variety of saturated fatty acids that affect satiety, digestion, and metabolism in a complete and complex fashion. Eliminating saturated fats from our diet amounts to playing a risky guessing game with our health.

---

1. Dale Bauman (Liberty Hyde Bailey Professor, Cornell University, Ithaca, New York). 2006., *Inform*. Vol. 17(5), pg. 277

CHAPTER 6

THE SCIENCE ABOUT ALL THE GOOD FATS: MONO, POLY, AND ESSENTIAL FATS AND THEIR BIOCHEMISTRY

Monounsaturated fatty acids (MUFAs)

Like the name implies, a monounsaturated fatty acid has one double bond (this is the fatty acid caterpillar that forgot one pair of shoes) and therefore bends easily. This bond is in the ninth position from the omega end, and so these fatty acids are also commonly called 'omega 9' fats. MUFAs are more dynamic than saturated fatty acids, and less stable when processed or heated, but they are *more* stable than polyunsaturated fatty acids. They have carbon chain lengths from 14-24 atoms long. Remember that the chain length of a fatty acid influences how fast it will metabolise, and that all fats have a combination of monounsaturated, saturated and polyunsaturated fatty acids in their make-up. No fat is purely monounsaturated. MUFAs have their place in a well balanced diet, but they are not complete enough in their nutritional functions to be the predominant source of dietary fat.

Despite the current belief paradigm that monounsaturated-rich fats such as olive, canola, safflower and sunflower oils are completely benign, they will in fact raise blood triglyceride levels, and interfere with the metabolism of the essential fatty acids linoleic and linolenic, if eaten too often or in too-great quantities. The monounsaturates have very diverse application as cooking oils, and are also present in many of the most popular processed and packaged foods we eat today. It is not hard to get enough monounsaturated fats into the diet, as they are plentiful and tasty and all around us.

Food and oil sources high in monounsaturated fatty acids

Most of these monounsaturated-rich oils and foods will also contain the *poly*unsaturated fatty acids omega 3 and 6, but in lower concentrations than omega 9. They are called monounsaturated fats because this is the *dominant* fatty acid type in these foods and oils. Use MUFA oils for fast stove top cooking, or blend them with quality saturated fat and use in baking. Always buy small bottles of a few different monounsaturated oils and use a variety throughout the week. Whatever quality one of these oils is missing, another is sure to have.

'Monousaturated' oils and their monounsaturated percentages

Olive oil	71%	Beef Tallow	48%
Avacado oil	60-71%	Peanut oil	48%
Canola oil	62%	Lard	44%
Filbert	69-81%	Palm oil	40%
Almond	61%	Salmon	37-49%
Eggs	50%	Cocoa Butter	34%
Chicken fat	49%	Butterfat	31%

These fats have higher Omega 6 and 3 fatty acids as well as Omega 9, which is listed.

Corn	28%	Sunflower oil	19%
Tuna	28%	Flaxseed oil	17%
Soybean oil	24%	Grape seed oil	16%
Walnut oil	23%	Safflower oil	13%
Cottonseed oil	20%	Human milk	36%

Canola oil is one of the most popular monounsaturated-rich oils in North America. It was first developed by means of induced mutation breeding, but subsequent technological advances led to genetically modified (GM) strains that account for most of the canola we use today. Early varieties of canola oil were called LEAR oil, which stands for 'low erucic acid rapeseed' oil. Canola is derived from the European rapeseed plant, which is a member of the mustard seed family. Rapeseed had a high (50%) erucic acid content; erucic acid is a long-chain monounsaturated fatty acid once believed to be toxic to humans, despite the fact that rapeseed oil has been widely used for centuries. For this reason erucic acid was mutated out of the rapeseed, and canola was developed. Europeans continue to use rapeseed oil. But the mutated/genetically-modified version, canola, which was created in Canada (hence the name- from CAnadian Oilseed, Low-Acid)) is preferred in North America. More recent research has disproved the assumption that erucic acid is toxic.

Advances in biochemistry, and in our understanding of plant genetics, have helped facilitate the genetic modification technologies that now make it possible to change the composition of fats more precisely than could ever be achieved through traditional plant breeding. Genes that control certain characteristics of oils are spliced into the DNA of those oils that have the most desirable traits. These genetic modifications are generally intended to create a fat whose composition and properties are optimised for commercial handling – and some say these foods are better for our health. Genetic modification is more often used to improve the yields of crops than to alter their fatty acid profiles. Herbicide-tolerant canola was being raised on about 3.0 million hectares of land worldwide in 2002 — part of an estimated total of 58.7 million hectares of land under GM crops.

Canola oil is a 'high oleic fat', containing 57-62 % oleic acid — the monounsaturated fatty acid with a double bond at carbon 9. This is the same fatty acid predominant in olive oil, from which it gets its name. The remainder of canola oil's profile comprises 23% omega 6 and 10-15% omega 3 (both polyunsaturated fats) and about 5% saturated fats. The fatty acid balance of omega 6 to omega 3 makes canola a relatively healthy product by today's mainstream standards. (See the ratios in the next section to learn more about the balance of fatty acids.) If you don't have a problem with genetically modified foods, then expeller pressed, non-solvent extracted canola is a good fat to use. If you are not keen on eating GM foods than canola oil should be avoided, expeller pressed or not. There is no such thing as 'organic' canola oil though I have seen oil advertised as such in products and health foods stores.

The original canola oil was 65 percent monounsaturated fat to 30 percent polyunsaturated fatty acids and 5 percent saturated. This made canola oil a most desirable product at the time of its début, since stories of the evils of saturated fats were already thoroughly entrenched in consumer consciousness. Canola was well-received, as the fat we had all been waiting for; it was stable enough for home cooking and hearty enough to tolerate some heat and processing in commercial applications, it had a good combination of omega 6 to omega 3 fatty acids and it had a minimal saturated fat content. It was hailed as the salvation of our North American arteries, resurrected from the imperfect rapeseed oil that nature had supplied us with for thousands of years. Hallelujah! North Americans started to oil up with canola! Manufactured food products like, chips, cookies, pastries and taco chips all got cooked up in monounsaturated canola oil. Canola displaced the saturated fat palm oil as the dominant oil in the North American diet.

Canola has continued to be modified since its original creation. One mutated version is a fat with a higher omega 9 content (the same properties as olive oil) and even lower omega 6 levels. This is a change that permits manufacturers to use it even more extensively in prepared foods, because of its more stable fatty acid configuration. This newer version can be heated longer and at higher temperatures without oxidizing. Other fats have followed in the footsteps of high-oleic canola; high-oleic safflower, sunflower, and even high oleic palm oil have become increasingly prevalent in manufactured foods. The high-oleic varieties can tolerate more heat than the original versions of all these fats. They range in concentration from75 to 79% oleic acid, and there is also a 'mid-oleic' 65% oleic acid sunflower oil. As production of these genetically modified fats becomes commonplace, in response to the needs of commercial food production, you can expect to find more and more of them on grocery store shelves, sold as products for use in high-heat domestic food preparation.

Once canola oil's monounsaturated omega 9 content was raised, it could be used for fried cooking, and processed into packaged food products with a long shelf life, because of the decreased risk of oxidation. There was no more need for saturated fats; monounsaturated canola would save us from the perils of heart disease. It has been nearly 25 years since the début of canola oil, and it is now ubiquitous. A survey of any grocery store would reveal that most packaged and prepared foods are loaded with canola oil. Both the high-oleic version and the original version can be found in every sort of food product under the sun. North Americans have managed handily to replace saturated fats with monounsaturated oils in every aspect of their diets. But it's not working for us; we still suffer high rates of heart disease, now joined by the more recent epidemics of diabetes and obesity.

Olive Oil

Olive oil is the Mediterranean's canola oil, without the genetic engineering. It has nourished cultures since the beginning of western civilization. The cultivation of olives and the making of olive oil is considered an art, and the quality of the oil from their farm or from their region is something that families take very seriously. When we go up to Zia Filomena's farm North of Toronto, Uncle Nick usually pulls out a fresh bottle of oil from Italy, generally brought back by the last person to have visited the old country. He'll pour it onto a spoon and glide it under our noses to let us savour the pure, sharp aroma. He always asks if I want to taste it, but I'm not quite there yet – taking oil by the spoonful. He licks his lips and drinks down the liquid gold, to prove its quality and goodness. And it is good. It will vary in colour, aroma, and flavour depending on when it was harvested, and whether the soil was pure or chemically enhanced, but most olive oil is extracted under strict laws governing temperature, the number of pressings, the quality of the olives used and oxygen exposure. All of these restrictions improve the quality of the resulting oil.

It is because of the regulations controlling olive oil's extraction that this monounsaturated oil maintains so many of its healthful qualities. A superior olive oil will be sold in an opaque bottle, will have a greenish hue and should be stored at a consistent temperature. I'd caution against buying the bulk (typically three litre) cans of oil for home use; this much oil will not be used fast enough to ensure that it retains its healthful properties. The large cans are meant for restaurants and facilities serving large numbers of people. If your supply of oil lasts longer than two months, it would be wise to buy it in smaller containers. Sixty years ago, when my husband was a small boy in Italy, olive oil was delivered daily by horse and buggy, just like we used to get milk delivered every morning. Oil in Italy was produced and sold by cottage industries that served the local community. Nona Santilli would send Paolo out into the street to chase the oil cart man and get his one-cup glass jar filled with a day's supply of oil. This system ensured the freshest, healthiest oil each and every day. Olive oil can be used for quick cooking on the stove-top under moderate heat, but not for extended periods. If it's cooked too long a foul odour will reveal that the oil is no longer good and should not be eaten. The rotten smell is the result of the fat breaking down, so proliferating free radicals that will damage our cells. When monounsaturated oil gets to this point any anti-oxidants that might have been in the oil will have perished. Any oil with this degree of degradation will wreak havoc on the cellular level.

The monounsaturated oil of the olive is a wonderful, nutritious fat, and it should be used daily in our diets. It does not 'compete' with other fats in healthfulness. It has its own merits, different from those inherent in the saturated fats of butter, lard, and tallow. It cannot be used to replace these fats. But *together* with butter, lard, and tallow, olive oil helps lay the foundations for quality, balanced nutrition.

Polyunsaturated fatty acids (PUFA) – The Essential Fatty Acids

The last two decades have witnessed a media bombardment of 'good fat' information, as 'good fats' became a tagline that identified the omega 3 and 6 fatty acids as different from all the other fats and fatty foods that had suffered such bad press for so long. It was strange to imagine that there might be fats that the body actually *needed* to survive and thrive. The public had been fed so many warnings about fats for so long that the concept of a fat that was beneficial to health took a bit of time to get used to.

Essential fatty acids are 'essential,' because, unlike most other fats, they cannot be manufactured in the body from other nutrients, and therefore must be obtained in food or by supplement. Deficiency symptoms have been strongly associated with such problems as forgetfulness, predisposition to Alzheimer's, arthritis, misbehaviour, moodiness, PMS, difficulty in learning, criminal activity, violence, suicide, vision loss, skin disorders, inflammatory conditions, heart disease, and failure to thrive — to list a few. This makes omega 6 and 3 EFAs sound a bit like modern day snake oils. But even if they're sold like like snake oil, the difference is that their benefits are real.

Information on essential fatty acids became more widely available in book stores (and eventually on the internet) during the late 1980s and through the 1990s. By 2003 the momentum had resulted in widespread demand for new food products containing the essential fats and their derivatives. Essential fatty acids became the most widely sold nutritional supplements. Now that consumers are convinced that these 'essential fats' should be part of a healthful diet, it would be beneficial to learn how, why, and in what proportions we need the omega 3 and 6 polyunsaturated essential fatty acids.

The following section offers an overview of the classification and structure of the fatty acids. I think it is important to include this information, even though it may seem excessive; changes to the quality of food labelling around trans fatty acids got a lot of attention when people started to understand their full implications for our health. The same is true of omega 6 and 3. If consumers can grasp some of the essential concepts of fat-related biochemistry, they will be in a better position to participate in the efforts required to change food policy and food choices. And the more often we are exposed to information the more familiar it will become. Don't be discouraged if this information seems way beyond your needs, or beyond what you feel you want to learn or are able to understand. Hopefully your subconscious will hold on to bits of it, so that when you come across the information again it will make more sense.

It seems to be a part of our North American mentality to want to wildly overstate the benefits or evils of a given food. If a little of something is deemed healthy, we have to believe that that more must be better!

And that even more is healthier still. Likewise if a food is deemed less than healthful, then abstaining from it altogether must be the 'healthiest' thing to do. This attitude has a lot to do with our ongoing contemporary struggle with ill health.

The Two Essential Fatty Acids

Linoleic Acid, Omega 6: abbreviated as 18:2w6. The 18 tells us the number of carbons in the fatty acid chain, 2 is the number of double bonds, (it forgot 2 pairs of shoes), and 6 is the position of the first double bond. 'Omega' means that the double bonds are 3 carbons away from the methyl end of the fatty acid (the end where the caterpillar attaches to the twig) rather than the carboxyl end. The fatty acids are all in a *cis* configuration. This term refers to the position of all the hydrogen atoms; they are on the same side and not opposite each other as in a *trans* fatty acid. This same-sided cis configuration makes the fatty acids capable of bending and moving easily. This flexibility affects the properties, behaviour, and functions of the oil in our body.

The main sources of omega 6 fatty acids are: corn oil, safflower oil, sunflower oil, soybean oil, mixed vegetable oil, and to a lesser extent canola oil, and sesame seeds, almonds, peanuts, brazil nuts, pistachios and their oils.

Alpha-Linolenic Acid, Omega 3: abbreviated 18:3w3. This fatty acid is similar to omega 6 but its fatty acids start on the *third* carbon from the methyl end, and it has one more double bond, initially, than omega 6 linoleic acid. The cis configuration is a prominent feature of the omega 3 fatty acid as well, so it too kinks and folds in and on top of itself, making it difficult for these fats to align. They will therefore not aggregate in the blood.

The main sources of omega 3 rich fats are: Flax seeds, flax seed oil, and fish. Hemp, pumpkin, soybean, walnut and dark-green leaves also have a bit of omega 3 coupled with a bit of omega 6 as well. Table 1 (below) gives the percentages of omega 6, and 3 fatty acid profiles.

Omega 3 and 6 fatty acids are very fragile fats. Because they have such high concentrations of double bonds they can oxidise and cause free radical damage very easily. The omega 3 rich fats and their derivatives have the lowest saturation point of any edible fats and are extremely sensitive to light, oxygen, and heat. For this reason they have to be stored in opaque bottles, their shelf-life is a paltry six to eight weeks after opening, and they *must* be stored in the fridge. This short shelf life was the reason omega fats were removed from food sources in the first place. Since I began writing this book the methodology for manufacturing omega fats into food products has changed and become more sophisticated. The shelf life for omega fats is still limited however, and affects how much and what concentration can be added to foods. Because of the fragility of omega 3 fats they should never be heated directly. They can be used on top of hot foods but not cooked.

Omega 3 and omega 6 fatty acid content of common foods and oils

Notice that all these fats below in the first list, except for the flax oil, have more O6 than O3. These are the oils that many health-conscious consumers are actively looking to increase in their diet, despite the fact that they have very low levels of omega 3 and very high levels of the omega 6 fatty acid that we are already consuming far too much of, as will be discussed at length in chapter 11.

TABLE 1

	Omega 3	Omega 6
Flax oil	58%	14%
Canola	7%	30%
Hemp	25%	55%
Pumpkin	15%	42%
Soybean oil	7%	54%
Walnut	5%	51%

The following foods and fats have even less omega 3 than those in the previous list. Their fatty acid profile has more omega 9, which is again coupled with a rich concentration of the omega 6 fatty acids. Most of these fats have been modified in recent years to increase their concentration of omega 9 and are referred to as 'high oleic' fats.

The Omega Fatty Acids in Commonly Used Unsaturated Oils

Food Oil	06 %	09 %	03 %
Safflower oil	77%	14%	0%
Sunflower oil	71%	16%	1%
Corn oil	57%	29%	1%
Soybean oil	54%	23%	8%
Walnut oil	54%	25%	11%
Cottonseed oil	54%	19%	2%
Peanut oil	33%	48%	0%
Canola oil	22%	61%	10%

Olive oil and flaxseed oil have unique combinations of fatty acids, quite different from those listed above:

Olive oil	10%	71%	1%
Flaxseed oil	17%	18%	55%

The foods in the following list are moderate in omega 3 linolenic acid but rich in the elongated forms of omega 3- DHA, docosahexaenoic acid and EPA, eicosapentaenoic acid. Plant algae is the only vegetarian source of these vital omega 3 fats; all other significant sources are fish – though there are moderate amounts in the eggs of flaxseed-fed hens.

EPA and DHA concentration

	EPA	DHA	EPA/DHA /3oz serving
Anchovy	.763	1.29	1.747
Sardine	.493	.590	.835
Tuna	1.141	.363	1.278
Cod	.103	.173	.235
Haddock	.076	.162	.202
Sea Bass	.206	.556	.648
Caviar	2.741	3.800	5.560
Salmon	.411	1.429	1.564
Herring	.909	1.105	1.172
Trout	.211	.265	.405
Bass	.305	.458	.649
Crustaceans	.295	.118	.351

Both essential fatty acids transfer oxygen. Not too many people know about the important role linoleic and linolenic oils play in respiration — transferring oxygen from the air in our lungs, through the thin lung membranes, through capillary walls and into the oxygen-binding haemoglobin in red blood cells, which then carries the oxygen to our cells. These fatty acids also hold the oxygen in our cell membranes, where together they act as an important barrier to foreign organisms that would otherwise enter cells and make us very sick. Throughout my years as an athlete and in coaching recreational runners I have always supplemented with omega 3 flaxseed oil, and encouraged others to do the same. I felt that I recovered from hard workouts faster when it was in my diet, and it did more good on long runs than the recommended carbohydrate diet.

The highly unsaturated oils have a high surface activity because of all those double bonds, and this enables them to act as carriers – transporting toxins to the body surface for excretion from the kidney, lungs, skin, and intestinal tract. The negative charge of the essential fats plays an important role in the production of *bio-electric currents,* which in turn are crucial to nerve, muscle, heart, and membrane functions, and the maintenance of natural body rhythms. No other fats within cell membranes do this.

Essential fats form a part of the structural cell membranes, just as saturated fats do. They help to keep the proteins in their place with the electrostatic attractive force of their double bonds. This electrostatic energy helps to control the movement of particles in and out of the cells, and when activated will generate currents that send messages to other cells. A well-functioning organism is all about communication: cells, organs, and systems all need to communicate with each other for bodily functions to maintain their rhythms and stay synchronized. Essential fats help increase the metabolic rate by making cell membranes more sensitive to insulin. The more receptive cells are to the hormone insulin, the more efficiently and effectively they will utilize sugar from the blood. So fat does benefit sugar and starch metabolism. Essential fats help increase muscle recovery by speeding up the conversion of lactic acid (the muscle stiffness you feel after a hard workout is the result of this by-product) to carbon dioxide and water. All foods should break down cleanly to carbon and hydrogen, free of toxic by-products. Omega 3 fats help achieve this.

Essential fats enhance the immune system by means of their effects on the inflammatory/anti- inflammatory pathways. A balanced and effective inflammatory/ anti-inflammatory process is critical for minimizing degenerative diseases such as arthritis, cardiovascular disease, diabetes, obesity, and fatty organ deposits. The inflammatory and anti-inflammatory pathways are both necessary for optimum health; and a properly balanced intake of omega 6 and 3 is a crucial part of achieving a healthy balance between the two.

Remember; if there is to be any abatement in inflammatory disorders such as arthritis, PMS, heart disease, asthma, and thrombosis, then omega 6 must be decreased in our diets, not increased.

CHAPTER 7
A TANGO WITH BUTTER

Butter and health

In 1910, North Americans were eating an average of 18 lbs of butter each per year. By 1950 butter consumption was down to 10 lbs, and from 1970 onwards it remained steady at 4.6 lbs per person per year. Newer statistics show that consumption is down again, to 4.2 lbs a year. North Americans are eating less butter than ever before in our history, but we're fatter than ever, and still dying of heart disease. And our heart attack rate began its increase pretty much as our consumption of butter started to decline. The myths about butter being bad for us have misled people long enough. There is no reason whatsoever to avoid butter any longer, and there never was. In fact, the opposite is true; avoiding butter can be hazardous to your health!

The fats in butter have specific benefits to human health. And for some of us, butter even benefits other aspects of human nature. (How about Marlon Brandon in *Last Tango in Paris!*). Butter has been an essential source of nutrition for many tundra-dwellers worldwide. People in more tropical regions tend to rely on other sources of saturated fat, but those of us in the cold were once raised, from gestation onwards, with all the benefits of butter. Stove-top frying was done with butter, warm vegetables were dressed in butter and toast was smothered in the stuff. Baking actually called for butter, there was a thick layer on the sandwiches in our lunch boxes, a dollop topped hot oatmeal, and it even made it into the occasional cup of hot tea on cold winter afternoons. Butter was once highly valued, and in most households it was used several times a day.

It was in the 1960s that the first whispers were heard about butter being bad for our health. Before then, people only replaced butter with margarine because of the difference in price; margarine was the economical alternative to butter. But by the mid 1970s margarine had become a secular religion. Butter was simply not to be used, unless you had a death wish. Margarine hip-checked butter right off the grocery store shelves.

Remember the margarine commercials that ran during The Waltons on television? (Remember John-Boy?) The plastic margarine container would lift its lid to tell us about all the merits of unsaturated fats, and contrast them with the dire hazards of eating butter. Kids all mimicked this commercial, running around and yelling, "tastes like butter but it's not". Children raised in the 1960s and 70s had the perils of saturated fat and butter etched right onto their view of the world. I have vivid memories of my skinny mother trying to sell the 'butter is bad' idea to my grandmother. I can still see the black and white linoleum tiles in Grandma's kitchen, the cast iron foot-peddle Singer sewing machine against the wall, and the deep white porcelain sink that always had a few tea-stained cups in it. Mom would shake her finger at Grams as Grams spread that delicious yellow gold onto small pieces of bread, then topped them with a teaspoon of jam. Grams would taunt my mother in her shaky voice: "Here you go Missy," she would say as she handed me the sweet, rich, deadly treat. "Mindy, do you want some jam and toast too?"

Grandma Doolittle wasn't buying into the 'butter is bad' con no matter how much skinny little Dorothy went on about its perils, and the need to use 'unsaturated' margarine in its place. Grams grew up on a farm in rural Quebec, and she inherently knew the value of real food. Her family drank their own cows' milk, collected the hens' eggs, slaughtered their own beef and hunted deer. They had cats not as pets but to catch the mice, and Grams learned the hard way that baby chicks need a real hen, not a little girl, to keep them warm. One night she put a dozen new chicks into her bed, and by morning she had rolled over all of them.

This story always mortified Mindy and me, but Grams was nonchalant about it, shaking her head with a bit of a giggle, because of course she'd learned the chicks hadn't needed her, they'd needed their real mother. Grams was a no-nonsense, trial-and-error autodidact. And one thing she'd learned was that no baby on that farm thrived without the right kind of good old fashioned fat and loving. (And a healthy dollop of faith didn't hurt either.) She only got to grade six before she was forced to stay home to help run the farm and care for her 12 brothers and sisters. Some of them died before the age of 5, but many of them thrived into their late 90s, like she did. No skinny thirty-something daughter was going to lecture her about healthy foods. I still love butter and jam in the afternoons.

Fatty acid profile of butter

Looking at a breakdown of butter's specific fatty acid profile makes clear the wide variety of fatty acids it contains. We'll see in detail later how the *combination* of fatty acid chain lengths is a very important issue that has so far largely been ignored.

Short chain fatty acids:

butyric acid	4c - 4%
caproic acid	6c - 2%
caprylic	8c - 1%
capric	10c - 3%

Medium chain fatty acids:

lauric	12c - 3%
myristic	14c - 11%
pentadecanoic	15c - 2%

Medium to long chain fatty acids:

palmitic	16c - 27%
margaric	17c - 1%

Long-chain fatty acids:

stearic	18c - 12%

Unsaturated fatty acids:

palmitoleic	16:1 - 2%
oleic	18:1 - 29%
linoleic	18:2 - 2%
linolenic	18:3 - 1%

Butter is rich in short, medium and long-chain fatty acids. The short and medium chain fatty acids make up 26% of butter's profile – that's a quarter! And more than a third of its fatty acid content is unsaturated. This is pretty much at odds with butter's crude classification as 'saturated fat'. The shorter chain components affect how butter metabolises, and play a major part in its overall affects on human health. Short and medium chain fatty acids metabolise quickly. They avoid being rearranged into micelles for transport in the blood, and they cannot aggregate in the blood or cause any harm when their first and only 'digestive destination' is the liver. The saturated fat stearic acid (12% of butter's total fatty acid profile) also has unique metabolic traits in that it converts automatically into the unsaturated fat oleic acid. Stearic acid, though classified as a saturate, has a neutral affect on blood lipids and cholesterol, and does not act like a saturated fat once in the body. None of the short-chain fatty acids, with their metabolic efficiency and their inability to aggregate, behave like true saturated fats. So we can see that 37% of butter is neutral saturated fat and 34% is unsaturated fats, and thus that 71% of the fat in butter has a benign affect on blood lipid profiles. So you be the judge; is butter bad?

The short-chain butyric acid of butter is essential for maintaining healthy intestinal flora, which help to keep digestion efficient and complete. One of the most important elements of good nutrition is efficient and thorough assimilation of nutrients from the digestive tract, and without a healthy balance of gut flora digestion will slow down and constipation will result, since this balance is essential for assimilating the nutrients that you ingest. If the good bacteria in the intestines do not have a source of fuel that enables them to flourish, then bad bacteria will overpower them.

And unfortunately, bad bacteria are always likely to have plenty of fuel, since they feed on the sugars that are so prevalent in our diets. Bad bacteria feed on any type of sugar, including refined sugar, brown sugar, broken down carbohydrates, high fructose corn syrup, honey, maple syrup…in short, anything! Bad bacteria overgrowth can lead to disorders like leaky gut syndrome, irritable bowel syndrome, colitis, candida albicans and (the one I see most often) carbohydrate cravings. The digestive system needs a balance of 'good' and 'bad' bacteria to ensure a well-maintained digestive system, and the bacteria need to be fed if they are going to stay alive and do their job.

The short-chain butyric and caproic acids in butter work as anti-fungals in the intestinal tract. As pointed out earlier, the lumen requires fuel to keep its cellular layer active, healthy and clean. These gut cells have a vital role to play in managing how other nutrients reach your body; they must have a source of food and protection. The digestive system needs direct nourishment and care. Butter's butyric and caproic acids help to do that job.

The butyric acid in butter also helps regulate cellular growth in the colon (the big intestine); it helps prevent bad cells from proliferating, by facilitating the programmed cell death known as *apoptosis* (think of it as 'popping' the head off a cell so it dies). Essentially, butyric acid is said to affect the 'expression' (the transformation of DNA information into functional parts of a cell) of genes in several types of cell. The apparent control of gene expression by butyric acid led researchers to suggest that these are tumor-suppressing behaviors, especially evolved for the colon. That's a big benefit from a little bit of daily butter. (Is colon cancer on the rise of late?)

More than a quarter – 27% – of the fat in butter is palmitic acid. *The heart muscle itself uses saturated palmitic acid as a preferred fuel.* Doesn't it seem strange that the very organ we are trying to protect with these extremely low saturated fat diets actually uses a saturated fat for its own fuel source? This says to me that perhaps there's more to saturated fats than meets the eye.

Butter is an excellent source of fat-soluble **vitamin A,** and the body needs 5,000 UI of vitamin A per day. It is needed for healthy vision, and it is used to lay down bone during growth, to help heal tissue after injury or surgery, and to protect against infection. Vitamin A stimulates the growth of the base layer of skin cells and all the mucous membranes of the nose, intestinal tract, respiratory lining and bladder. Vitamin A's role in maintaining healthy mucous membranes involves helping to fight off infections from inside and outside the body. We put on sunscreen to protect our outer skin from the sun; think of vitamin A as a cream for the inside layers of 'skin'. Vitamin A keeps the epithelial cells of the digestive system and the respiratory system healthy.

Vitamin A is used by the adrenal glands and the thyroid gland for metabolism. Together the thyroid and adrenals contribute to the health of the cardiovascular system. Vitamin A is always one of the most essential nutrients in a developing nation's food supply because of its strong immune enhancing role. Vitamin A is a potent antioxidant at levels above 10,000 UI per day. The average American diet takes in just 4,000 UI daily, which forces the body to use stored vitamin A from the liver, fat tissue, eye, lungs and kidneys. Taking vitamin A out of storage requires the use of the mineral zinc. Our diet should not make it necessary for our body to tap into its stored supplies of nutrients; these should be reserved for times of infection and stress, not simply for making up an ongoing nutrient deficiency, and a diet low in saturated fat can easily be deficient in vitamin A. Along with the vitamin D also found in butter, vitamin A performs an essential role in the absorption of calcium, which as we know helps to build and maintain strong bones and teeth.

In the winter of 2007 the media jumped on the promotional bandwagon for vitamin D, which is activated by exposure to the sun. Getting enough vitamin D can be a real issue for people living in colder climates where sunshine is limited. But there was no mention, among all the hype for sunshine, that vitamin D can be obtained from dairy products, including butter. The official message is so convoluted; remove fat from your foods, eat only low-fat versions of everything, then supplement your diet with the nutrients found in fatty food! And vitamins A and D are both fat-soluble; even if you take them in supplement form, you have to eat fat to be able to assimilate them. Butter is also rich in the antioxidants vitamin E, selenium and cholesterol. (*Yes, cholesterol is an antioxidant!*) And because butter has a lot of saturated fatty acids, there is less oxidation — meaning the body's stored supply of vitamin E is not depleted, and will be on hand when needed to neutralize the oxidation of *unsaturated* fats like safflower, corn, soybean, and sunflower oils.

Conjugated linoleic acid, or CLA, is a vital nutrient that has been associated with such beneficial health effects as weight loss, enhanced immunity, protection against cancer and heart disease and increased bone mineralization. But there are fewer and fewer sources in our modern diets. CLA is a fatty acid. *Conjugated* refers to the pattern of alternating single and double bonds between carbon molecules that was once found in abundance in dairy products, and in the meat of cattle and wild game that grazed on fresh grasses and clover. It is not present in grains, fish, or poultry. Cows have the ability to 'conjugate' regular unsaturated fats like safflower oil in the rumen. Then this newly created fatty acid goes off to storage, and is used at the muscle level or in milk production. Supplementing cattle feed with safflower or soybean oil to increase the concentration of CLA is one of the latest animal science menu changes. Cows grazed in open pasture can also have exceptionally high levels of this conjugated fatty acid.

CLA has lately been the darling of the nutritional supplement industry, and a great deal of research has been going into its affect on health, in particular its relationship to weight loss. The studies are inconclusive, and little consensus has been reached yet regarding the impact of CLA in the diet. What studies do show is that on some level CLA is boosting metabolism at doses of 3-5 grams per day. That's a lot of gel capsules to consume without knowing what other biochemical processes might be affected (i.e, what the side-effects might be). Of course, CLA is also available in its natural form from wholesome, natural sources, but only foods with fat. So buying low fat dairy and lean cuts of meat will deny you the metabolic benefits of conjugated linoleic acid.

CLA can take several different forms, depending on where the double bond is positioned and where the cis and trans positions occur. So far the consensus among producers and consumers of supplements has been for the cis 9 trans 11 CLA. We can't control what the cow will manufacture (well, we can... but that's another story) but you can ensure that you get a dose or two of CLA most days with some form of fat from butter, beef or dairy. If you avoid saturated fats it will be difficult to get CLA, since your stomach can't manufacture it from sunflower oil like a cow's does. In the case of CLA, as with so many other nutrients, what we are currently experiencing are the *unforeseen consequences, for our metabolism as a whole, of the elimination of an entire category of food from our diet.* Those little doses of nutrients that seemed to be of little significance thirty years ago are now increasingly being recognised as essential for optimum health.

Butter also contains *lecithin,* an emulsifier of fats. Emulsifiers act to help blend water and oils together. Mother Nature has been so prescient; she has put things like lecithin right in the fatty foods that we might just need a little help to digest. Clever girl, that Mother Nature. Lecithin is also a constituent of bile acid, and of course bile helps to emulsify fats and prepare them for digestion. The phospholipids of lecithin are important in the structures of all cell membranes and healthy nerves. Lecithin can be bought as a supplement, but don't be fooled by the soy-based lecithin; it is a cheaper, highly processed product that cannot match the effectiveness of animal based lecithin. Lecithin should be eaten, as should most things, the way nature intended – as a part of their natural source. Lecithin is also found in eggs, and soybeans. A little bit of lecithin each day would go a long way towards improving our health.

Lung surfactant is the fluid encasing the alveoli in our lungs, and it serves the rather important function of allowing the lungs to stretch freely and to contract without collapsing. Lung surfactant is predominantly a saturated fat. It has to be said that it is 'predominantly' saturated because while it is biologically *supposed* to be a saturated fat, a diet that is high in other fats will result in the phospholipids of the lungs incorporating these fats as well. This substitution is believed to compromise the efficiency of the lungs.

Butter has *cholesterol!* Yes indeed it does. 20 mg per 2 teaspoon! The human body only absorbs about half of the cholesterol it takes in, which means that one serving of butter means a 10mg dose of cholesterol. *Oh No!!* But wait....one of the most important uses of cholesterol is as an anti-oxidant, controlling the free radical damage caused by unstable molecules from unsaturated oils. A healthy daily intake of butter serves to protect against this free radical activity. To say that the cholesterol in butter has a negative impact on one's health is ludicrous. In fact, in March 1991 Nutrition Week published a study showing that men who ate butter had *less* heart disease than men who ate margarine. Despite the well-known biochemistry of butter metabolism, and the fact that it is clearly harmless to arteries, butter continues to be one of the foods most regularly recommended for elimination from our diets in the name of good health. I believe this represents a grave error on the part of our policy makers; butter is not the culprit, or even an accessory, in the assault on our health.

". . The advice to reduce all saturated fat in the diet, which led to the increase use of hydrogenated vegetable oil, was rash advice that spawned problems. It turned out to be one of the worst things one could recommend... There is such a risk factor for coronary heart disease in switching from butter to margarines."[2]

Short-chain fats like butter and goat fat *do not contribute significantly to blood lipoprotein levels!* Short-chain fatty acids have no cholesterol-raising properties. Short-chain fats are not deposited in adipose tissue (fat on your body) and they are readily absorbed in conditions where the ability to absorb of long-chain fatty acids may be impaired. This means that short-chain fats and long-chain *saturated* fats may be used more efficiently and metabolized more cleanly than long-chain *unsaturated* fatty acids.

By avoiding saturated fats consumers have lost out on the vital health benefits that saturated fatty acids can provide. Replacing saturated fats with monounsaturated and polyunsaturated fats in order to lower blood cholesterol and help the heart is a completely misguided enterprise, and the campaign encouraging this shift in eating habits is noteworthy for its use of half-truths based on half-understood science. This approach to preventative healthcare only compromises our health in other ways.

To summarise: the butyric acid found in butter is a saturated fatty acid and it helps to maintain intestinal integrity, which improves digestion. The caproic acid in butter is a potent anti-fungal that penetrates the membranes of candida cells and breaks them apart, hindering the yeast's ability to replicate and preventing candida overgrowth. Palmitic acid, 27% of butter's profile, is the fuel of choice of the heart muscle, and our precious lung surfactant is made up of saturated fatty acids. Short-chain fats have been *proven* benign in their affect on heart disease and cholesterol levels. Short-chain fats are far too active to be stored in fat tissue on hips, bums, and thighs; they are not part of adipose tissue. Butter is a natural source of conjugated linoleic acid, a nutrient important in the metabolising of fat, while the lecithin in butter is an important emulsifier of fats. Butter's vitamin A and vitamin D contribute to immunity and to bone health. And butter is rich in anti-oxidants, vital for neutralizing the negative affects of oxidation. It is high time we restored this delicious, all natural, liquid gold to its place of pride in our diets! Go ahead – tango with butter.

---

2.   Dale Bauman. 2006. *Inform*. Vol. 17(5), pg. 277

CHAPTER 8

LARD, COCONUT AND PALM OIL

For the love of lard!

Lard and tallow consumption at the turn of the century was 12 pounds per person per year and heart disease accounted for 8% of deaths. Today, we consume less than 6.4 pounds per person per year, while heart disease is responsible for 46% of all deaths. It can't be the lard!

The fatty acid profile of Lard:

Lard is 58% unsaturated fat!

Medium chain saturated fatty acids:
Myristic acid with 14carbons, 2%

Long-chain saturated fatty acids:
palmitic acid with 16carbons, 26%
stearic acid with 18carbons, 14%

Monounsaturated fatty acids:
palmitoleic acid 18:1, 3%
oleic acid 18:2, 44%
gadoleic acid 20:1, 1%

Polyunsaturated fatty acids:
linoleic acid 18:2, 10%

Does anyone ever cook with lard any more? I have fond memories of weekends spent at Grandma Doolittle's. She always had a big glass jam jar on the counter top where she saved all the fat she drained from cooking. Once she'd poured it from the pan to the jar, it would harden into a sandy coloured solid. Sometimes, for a treat, she would toast a slice of bread and cover it with a generous serving of that countertop lard. I always refused this delicacy; her candy bowl, now adorning my desk, was always full of far more appetising options for a seven year old. Grandma Doolittle lived to be 96 years old, sprightly and agile as long as I can remember.

Lots of people nowadays don't even know what lard is! Lard is a rendered fat from pigs – as opposed to an non-rendered fat like suet. Lard was used for centuries here in North America, right up until the mid 1980s, when consumer health advocates rallied to have it practically eliminated from our food supply and replaced with hydrogenated vegetable shortenings. At that time hydrogenation wasn't even mentioned on food labels or packaging, and consumers had no idea of its prevalence – and no idea why they might want to know. Food policy makers endorsed its use, apparently unaware of its real biochemical significance. To the mass of consumers hydrogenated fat was presented as the desirable, unsaturated alternative to animal fat. French fries will never taste the same!

Stearic acid is a long-chain saturated fatty acid that is abundant in most meats and animal fats. Once in the body, stearic acid is converted to monounsaturated fatty acid. Stearic acid, despite all the bad press, is known to have a neutral affect on cholesterol profiles. It makes up about 14% of the fat content of lard.

It's inappropriate to label lard as a saturated fat, since in many ways it behaves more like an unsaturated fat – though it can be cooked at higher temperatures than unsaturated fats. It is hard at room temperature, but 58% of lard is unsaturated fatty acids. It has to be handled properly because its high unsaturated fat content means it can become rancid just like the other unsaturated fats. Lard is a versatile fat, in that it can come in soft smooth or hard forms, which have different properties and different uses. It is also rich in the antioxidants tocopherol and tocotrienols, and the 2-3% palmitoleic acid content of lard is valuable for its anti-microbial properties in the gut. So go ahead and spread it on toast if you are so inclined. But for Lord's sake stop pouring it down the drain, and running the hot water to keep it from plugging the pipes. My grandmother always hated it when my mother did that.

Merits of Lard

- Lard tolerates high heats without burning. This means it is a stable fat, even with cooking – producing fewer free radicals and so requiring fewer antioxidants from our bodies' stored supplies. North Americans are currently in a state of antioxidant deficiency as a result of our refined food diet, and this makes stability an important quality of fats .

- Lard is completely natural, without any colour, flavouring, additives, or binders, and no chemicals are used in it processing. We are learning more and more every year about the hazards of the chemical by-products used in processing our food supply. Using a little lard in place of refined unsaturated oils eliminates another source of potential hazards.

- Lard is a cooking fat, and used alongside other natural fats it should be seen as an essential food product, especially in colder climates.

- Lard is rich in vitamin D, which is essential for the absorption of minerals – particularly calcium and magnesium, the two bone-building minerals.

- Vitamin E, beta sistosterol and beta carotene are potent antioxidants that are refined out of the unsaturated oils. Lard provides plenty of these.

These merits are largely ignored, just like those of butter; further evidence that there is more to the story of saturated fats than the health conscience consumer will hear from official sources. Lard is only 28% saturated, and the labelling of it as a deleterious saturated fat has to be revisited. Our consumption of lard and other animal fats has decreased by more than 50% since the turn of the last century, while heart disease has increased by a similar proportion. Food for thought.

Coconut Oil

It seems like we've been warned against foods made with saturated coconut oil almost forever. Since the 1970s coconut oil has been systematically removed from our snack foods, fast foods and packaged foods. These were not the best places to get our coconut oil, but at least it was around, and there was a very logical reason for using it in those products, the details of which are covered in the chapter on oxidation. Here is the fatty acid profile of coconut oil:

Short chain saturated fatty acids:
Caproic acid with 6 carbons - 1%
Caprylic acid with 8 carbons - 8%
Capric acid with 10 carbons - 6%

Medium chain saturated fatty acids:
Lauric acid with 12 carbons - 47%
Myristic acid with 14 carbons - 18%

Long chain saturated fatty acids:
Palmitic acid with 16 carbons - 9%
Stearic acid with 18 carbons - 34%
Arachidic with 20 carbons - 1%

Unsaturated fatty acid:
8% total unsaturates

In the last several years quality coconut oil has enjoyed a resurgence. Perhaps this is because of the Asian influence on our diets and our cities, or perhaps savvy, health-conscious consumers have begun to undergo a paradigm shift away from unsaturated fats. Whatever the reason, coconut oil is now more widely available. As with all fats, organic, virgin varieties are the most healthful. Pesticides and herbicides are fat-soluble, and therefore coconuts that are sprayed with them will likely contain large residues, which will survive in coconut products. 92% of coconut oil is saturated. That means less than 8% of coconut oil is unsaturated. But 47% of coconut oil's fatty acids are 12 carbons long, and 18% are 14 carbons long; these fatty acids are medium in length, and *cannot* aggregate in the blood, despite being saturated fats, and therefore sharing a reputation as 'blood thickeners'. As was explained in the short chain saturated fat section, short and medium chain fats do not use bile or the liver for digestion. *The Chain length of a fatty acid, and how it metabolises, will affect our health more than its saturation point will.*

Unsaturated oils have up to 96% of their fatty acids in the form of long chain fatty acids, 18 carbons or greater. The long chain fatty acids from unsaturated vegetable oils such as safflower, sunflower, soybean, corn, and canola have a higher concentration of *calories*, ounce for ounce, than the mixed chain length saturated fats in butter, coconut, lard, and tallow. The difference is only about 100 calories per pound, but manufactured foods such as French fries, doughnuts, cookies, crackers and chips must contain far greater amounts of unsaturated oil in order to replicate the taste and texture of a tropical oil. And the same is true of packaged health food products. The end result is that manufactured food products such as cookies and crackers that are made with unsaturated fats are 2-3% *higher* in calories than if coconut or palm oil were used. There *are* companies like Voortman's who are still making cookies with butter, coconut and palm oil. Feel free to have two.

Coconut oil has many health enhancing properties besides its lower caloric value. The medium chain *lauric acid* in coconut oil has anti-microbial properties; lauric acid will penetrate a microbe in the gut and literally force the dangerous offender to burst, rendering it benign. The gut (or digestive tract, or *lumen*) is actually outside the body, and this fact involves numerous risks. Think of the intestinal track as a garden hose coiled inside the abdominal cavity, transporting food and nutrients from mouth to anus. The *outside* of the intestinal garden hose is integrated with the other organs and systems of the body, but the *inside* is separate from the rest of the abdominal cavity; this is the outside, inside of us. Food from the outside world is presented to the intestinal lumen before it is ready for the blood, which carries nutrients to the rest of the body. It is because of this that the lumen needs extra protection. The cells of the lumen have to be strong and to replicate efficiently, and they have to be able to ward off potential harm. Any food with anti-microbial properties is a wonderful and necessary part of a healthy diet. Coconut's lauric acid can help out in a big way.

Coconut oil is perfect for all high-heat cooking; it can be used in the oven, on the stove top, in commercial frying or deep-frying. It is stable and will resist oxidation up to 325°. It won't break apart and cause free radical damage like the unsaturated oils that are presently being used in its place. Coconut oil has an abundance of short chain saturated fatty acids that do not require digestion through the liver. These fatty acids, we know, do not require bile nor are they packaged into chylomicrons –

the suitcases in which fat is carried through intestinal walls and prepared for transport in the blood. The short chain saturates of coconut oil are largely used as a source of energy, just like a starchy potato, and sports enthusiasts and health-conscious eaters will both find coconut oil a very beneficial addition to their diet. Coconut oil metabolises like a starch for energy but it still satiates like only a saturated fat can, and it brings a load of nutrients with each serving as well. Coconut oil out-performs pasta for any endurance athlete.

It can be difficult to know how to use coconut oil, since it has been banished from our grocery stores. Store coconut oil on a shelf away from direct heat. It will melt and re-harden with fluctuations in room temperature. (Try to minimize these temperature fluctuations for your oil.) Coconut can be used for cooking things as varied as popcorn, stir-fries or shrimp, and it can replace vegetable oil in muffin mixes at a half or third the amount the recipe calls for. It does have a flavour that you might initially find odd if you have been predominantly using refined vegetable oils. But it tastes wonderful – just like fat should.

To make sure I get my serving of coconut oil daily I do these two things. About mid-afternoon when I have three more clients to see and I don't have time to eat, I have a cup of green tea with a dollop of coconut oil. If I have made a small two-cup pot of tea I mix raw honey with the organic coconut and drop it into the teapot. This is a highly nutritious and satisfying drink; it decreases the desire for food between meals and provides a healthy portion of enzymes and short chain fats. I love to be hungry for a meal, so not eating between meals is a bit of a sacrament for me. If the day gets longer than expected this little drink helps a lot. I also mix a tablespoon of coconut oil into blender drinks made with fruit, kefir, water, and protein supplement. This is a great meal on the run when I have a class at six o'clock at night and can't make it home for a proper dinner. My husband thinks it is absolutely ludicrous that I schedule myself to the point where I don't have time for a proper meal; this goes against all his Italian sensibilities. But when I do over-schedule, this power meal works really well. Oh, and I also rub coconut oil all over my body as a winter moisturizer when I get out of the shower. I never ever use commercial body creams. Coconut oil goes well in hot oatmeal, or mixed with butter for stove top frying, or just about anywhere you need a solid fat.

There has been an interesting coconut oil-related phenomenon at my office. I made sure not to tell my clients what to expect, and they still came back to me one after another to rave about the same phenomenon – the improved condition of their feet. (These are all women who get professional pedicures regularly, so they know their feet.) After consuming coconut oil on a regular basis, they all found that their heel calluses had vanished completely. Everyone's scalps were healthier and smoother, and the few women who had suffered from dandruff had none. One woman stopped taking coconut oil over the summer break to see what would happen; in September she went back to having her coconut tea after her rough heels returned.

I have never seen anyone put on weight from adding a little coconut oil to a healthy diet. It is so packed full of nutrients that it functions to drive the metabolism, not bog it down. Personally I always feel better with coconut oil as part of my daily routine. And don't forget that coconut milk is just as nutritious as the oil; use it in soup bases, blender drinks, porridge, hot cocoa and stir-fries. Organic shredded coconut can be added to just about anything, and when you get into the habit of using it once or twice a day, by week's end you will have treated yourself to a lot of great nutrients that otherwise would have been hard to accumulate.

Palm oil: a long chain 'saturate'

Palm oil and palm kernel oil are derived from the fruit of palm trees generally called 'oil palms'. Here is the fatty acid profile of palm oil:

Long chain saturated fatty acids:
   Myristic acid with 14 carbons - 1%
   Palmitic acid with 16 carbons - 45%
   Stearic acid with 18 carbons - 4%

Long chain unsaturated fatty acids:
   Oleic acid with 18 carbons monounsaturate - 40%
   Linoleic acid with 18 carbons polyunsaturate - 10%

Palmitic acid is a 16 carbon long fatty acid; it is a very colourful red-orange hue, and rich in anti-oxidants. Palm oil is known to have high concentrations of the antioxidant vitamin E's tocopherols and to-cotrienols, and of beta carotene, the precursor to vitamin A. And palm oil is rich in the complete form of vitamin A, an immunity enhancing vitamin, as well as flavones, squalene, and co-enzyme Q — which is a known essential antioxidant specifically for the heart. It has been used for over 5000 years in parts of the world where the palm tree thrives which is a real testament to palm oil's healthfulness. Palm oil, despite all its bad press, is difficult to implicate as a direct cause of heart disease, since its fatty acid profile is equal parts saturated and unsaturated fats. And the cultures that use palm oil as their primary fat source do not have heart disease rates nearly as high as those in North America.

Palm oil is not to be confused with palm *kernel* oil; the latter is found in the *nut* of the fruit, not in the fruit itself. Palm kernel oil is very similar to coconut oil in that its predominant (48%) fatty acid is the medium chain 12 carbon lauric acid. Recall the metabolic qualities of lauric acid discussed in the section on coconut oil, and the anti-microbial properties that it possesses. Palm kernel oil has merits that cannot be duplicated by any of the unsaturated fats that have come to replace it in our food supply. Look for it when (if?) you shop for processed foods; it is far more stable, has a naturally longer shelf life, and is less processed than vegetable oils.

If you are going to eat manufactured goods with fat in them this is the fat to choose.

The campaign against palm oil has been ongoing for decades, but it intensified in 1984, when food manufacturers and fast food restaurants began to be required by law to replace palm oil with other, unsaturated oils. Because part of its fatty acid profile was saturated, the powers-that-be decided that palm oil should be categorised as an unnecessary, un-healthy 'saturated fat'. The media were suddenly full of advertisements that claimed palm oil was 'poisoning' North Americans, despite the fact that palm oil represented no more than 1% of the edible fats in consumer diets. This campaign had a profound affect on the image of palm oil in North America, and was responsible for the introduction of unsaturated oils into processes in which stable saturated fats would normally have been used, such as high heat fryers and processed foods. And fryers across the continent have been using safflower, sunflower, cottonseed, and soybean oil ever since.

Diabetes and obesity rates started to rise steadily, taking their toll on the lives of North American children, teens, and adults, shortly *after* this mandated change away from palm oil. And yet here we are today; frying our French fries in safflower oil and baking our kids cookies full of polyunsaturated vegetable oils. I wonder if these oils will nourish hu-manity for another 5000 years!

CHAPTER 9
SATURATED FAT FOR HEALTHY KIDS

Poor little rich girls

As you've probably gathered by now, this book is arguing that we have been subjected to a steady stream of misinformation about the fats in our diet over the past forty years. Intended to safeguard our health, this misinformation has instead done it considerable harm.

And this contradiction is clearest and most problematic where it involves the health of our children. Here is a story that illustrates it perfectly. A prominent woman, whose husband is the CEO of an international clothing and lifestyles company, came to me for advice about her two small girls, five and seven years old. She was concerned about their lack of enthusiasm for school, and even for play. She explained to me that they were often tired and disinterested in the almost unlimited resources they had at their disposal; horse riding, ballet lessons, gymnastics lessons, skiing, water sports were all theirs for the asking. She was a very good mother, and only wanted her girls to be happy and engaged. But they just didn't seem to be. Their mother was a long-time enthusiast of yoga and healthy living, and she thought that perhaps an overhaul of the girls' diet might help them feel more energetic and happy, as they certainly should have been. The mother was convinced that the girls were eating well, but she was eager to explore potential nutritional deficiencies. She herself had always been "health conscious" and had never needed to diet. She was fit, trim, and as petite as ever.

I asked her, "Please describe what the girls eat on a typical school day, from early morning until bedtime, and include all their activities during the day as well." I wrote down her thoughts as she described a typical day in the life of her girls. "Well...they always eat a good breakfast", she stated proudly. "Usually cold cereal with skim milk."

"What kind of cereal?" I asked.

"They like Special K, that would be their favourite of the ones I buy."

"How do you choose your cereals?"

"Oh, usually by the amount of fat in a serving," she responded inno-cently. Hmmm. Well I suppose that by this measure Special K is one of the best choices, since it has only a meagre .1 grams of fat per 21 gram serving....*a tenth of a gram*! That is less fat than you'll find in most nat-ural whole grains!   The Q&A session moved on to the typical lunch the children were fed. It turned out that they liked baby carrots, and cucum-ber circles, and apple slices. They didn't always eat the low-fat yoghurt, and the cottage cheese usually came back in the lunch-box. They would always eat their deli ham sandwich – one or two slices of ham on whole wheat bread with mustard.

"Don't you put butter on the bread?"

"No. I think that butter on bread is just a conditioned habit."

Dinners for the girls was a hit and miss affair. Again they would gob-ble up their vegetables, but usually picked at their fish, or chicken, or slab of lean meat. They always ate dinner immediately after school, after which the nanny got them ready for bed while the parents ate *their* evening meal. For a nutritionist, information about daily habits and lifestyle is as vital as a record of the food her clients eat. We don't just see people in terms of the biochemical properties of the food that they eat; through experience we have also learned to recognise the quirky habits that have propelled our nation, one family at a time, into an epi-demic of obesity. And the diet of these girls reflected a lot of quirky habits. Here was the clincher: "What kind of bedtime snacks do the girls like to have?"

"Oh I don't give them food before bed. " The mother replied. "I just don't want them to develop bad habits!"

   Bad habits!! Since when is food a 'bad habit' for a child? I had to laugh and lighten the mood, otherwise I would have cried. "Mrs. X," I stated; "you are starving your girls! They need calories; they need fat; they even need a little bit of sugar to avoid creating the eating disorders that come from denial of foods. They need to eat protein and fat before bed in order to secrete the growth hormone that helps them grow and re-pair muscles. When they are fed at 4:30 pm and don't get a bedtime snack they go 15 hours without a morsel of food. Every day! We would all be pin-thin if we were food-restricted like that."

This is a clear example of a distorted nutrition belief. Diet recommendations for adults do not seamlessly apply to children as well. Restricted diets for children will result in poor health: malaise; irritability; moodiness; poor growth; poor digestion; tooth decay...the list goes on and on. Though I never met these little girls, their mother and I had several more appointments. Mrs. X decided that she would keep a confidential food journal on behalf of the girls. She would casually ask them how they enjoyed their meals and snacks. Her guidelines for the girls would start to incorporate snacks dense in protein and fat before bed, in portions appropriate for the little girls' sizes; things like peanut butter on pita or whole grain crackers, home-made coconut muffins, cheese and apple, or warm coconut milk. Butter, real mayonnaise, full fat organic yoghurt and milk became staples in the girls' diets. No more skim milk dairy products for these children. They started to enjoy flavourful regular-fat meat for dinner, all prepared in creative ways that would appeal to children. After three weeks they were much improved, and after six weeks Mom could no longer keep up with her little bundles of energy and enthusiasm.

Healthy eating- it's not rocket science

As a society we have become very much removed from our primordial nutritional needs. Confusion about nutritional needs has permeated all social classes and all ethnic cultures in North America. Obesity is more prevalent among lower socio-economic classes; and osteoporosis most prevalent among the white middle classes – and both of these diseases are closely related to poor nutrition. Vegetarian and religious groups fight with McDonald's about tallow in frying oil, seemingly unaware that using unsaturated oils for frying is a known health hazard, and hippy parents raise babies on strict, unnatural vegetarian diets not found in any traditional culture around the world. Nutrition confusion pervades all of modern society. Perhaps we had the answer a century ago, and just need to go full circle and return to our roots and the whole, hearty nutrition our ancestors enjoyed, just like Grandma Doolittle always maintained. In the example I've recounted, even a mother's instinct couldn't overcome the dictates of 'authoritative' nutrition misinformation from government and media – and her experience is all too typical. In our land of plenty we are generally quite poorly nourished. It is not necessary to eat low fat, no fat, or newfangled 'health' foods. And we should especially not be incorporating these products into the diets of our children. Saturated fat is essential for proper metabolism, and for the health of mind and body. To take the fat out of dairy foods is to take out the life force. Our children will not grow without adequate fat, their brains will not develop to potential, and they will end up as sickly adults.

I became a mother at 35. It was a violent five-hour natural birth with the aid of a calm midwife. It was also the most gruelling physical experience I had ever endured, surpassing any pain or physical demand that I could have ever imagined as an athlete. But as for all new mothers, it was the most important event in my life. As soon as I knew I was pregnant, I wanted to do everything right to ensure optimal health for Lucy (I just knew she was a girl). For the first time in my life I craved red meat. I didn't resist, and my husband, who is a chef, would season my steak then grind it up – because I wasn't used to cutting meat for a meal. Sounds absolutely juvenile, and it was! But my childhood likes and dislikes governed my food choices as an adult. I was sure red meat was something I wouldn't like, even if I was craving it....and the urge to eat it was so strong I would have hunted it down if I'd had to! After two weeks of copious calorie intake, I'd already gained the first 8 pounds my body needed. During my pregnancy I ate even more fat than I'd been eating already. I ate steak, French fries, enormous sticky buns... sometimes two in one sitting. I ate cheese with a spot of wine from time to time, and vegetables by the plateful, covered in pats of butter. And I never felt full. At the end of the nine months I had gone from 108 to 134 pounds. My husband Paolo matched my weight gain pound per pound.

Lucy was 6 pounds 14 ounces at birth, and I think for the first two days I lay awake just to look at her as she slept. As our tiny child grew, and grew, and grew, I no longer stayed awake to marvel at her, but slept whenever I could! She gained weight so rapidly that I used to weigh her at the produce store on their vegetable scale. By the time she was 10 months all her teeth were in, far ahead of schedule. Paolo took over the feeding responsibilities with joy, because I just couldn't stand the mess. Who knew that one little person could make so much mess with one bowl of food? Paolo's love of culinary art was seeping into Lucy by osmosis, and she ate all the spices he minced into her puréed food. Paolo gave her whole salmon, tuna, sardines – with garlic, parsley, pepper, and lemon on everything. We puréed grass-fed beef. One day Lucy was in her high chair, yelling orders in a broken baby babble as Paolo scurried around the kitchen. To help with the chaos I took the 6-ounce medallion of steak and started to cut it into baby-sized slices for her. I was convinced that because of its colour and texture she would refuse meat once it was no longer puréed for her. To my utter surprise, she banged the fat little fist holding her miniature Winnie the Pooh fork onto the high-chair tray and yelled in her most dictatorial little voice: "No cut, no cut, and no cut!!" I froze, then composed myself and plopped the steak right onto her high-chair tray. Those two little hands took hold of the steak, one on each side, and she raised it to her mouth and tore at it like a sabre-toothed tiger. I stood in stunned silence as she savagely devoured 6 ounces of tender red meat without once throwing it across the room. She flushed it down with a baby bottle of water and slept, and slept, and slept.

The lesson was so clear to me. I realized that I too imposed my own culinary quirks onto my child; and I should have been so much more aware. I believe our children are not born junk-food addicts; this is something they are taught. Given a well-rounded diet on a weekly cycle children will cheerfully adapt balanced eating habits. Even as a nutritionist I don't abstain from any foods myself, or deny them to Lucy. She has as much access to Nutella, candies and truffles as she does to fruit, vegetables, cold meat, milk, and juice. It's been a fascinating experiment to play a part in her developing food habits. I've learned that all the asking and begging and demanding around junk food is more about winning the argument than it is about the junk itself. She's astute at remembering what foods cause reactions for her. She has taught herself that two tubs of yoghurt in one sitting will give her throat a hairball, and that coloured candies make her feel agitated, or as she would describe it, "jumpy". Too much chocolate feels 'funny', and too much watermelon feels "way too full." There is joy around food; it's how Papa cares for us, and it's something we celebrate. Every meal we mention the ripeness of the tomatoes or the sharpness of the meat. Lucy has to try everything that is served, at least once, "Because," as Lucy herself observed, "we never know, that even our taste buds grow and maybe we actually do like something but only think that we don't." I believe that if we want our children to be healthy we have to set a healthy example. So prepare foods differently, spice things differently... if we expand our own culinary horizons, those of our children will follow.

Fat for growth

Michael Gurr is a biologist who for decades has written for a journal called *Lipid Technology.* He has amalgamated a great many of his articles into a textbook entitled *Lipids in Nutrition and Health: A Reappraisal* – including an excellent comparative study demonstrating the effects of fat on growth. (See the bibliography at the back of the book for a full reference to Gurr's work.) The book includes a study that records Gurr's assessment of the growth of rats, and the development of their internal organs, when the rats were fed a variety of restricted diets, each limited to a single specific food. The effects of this nutrient-specific diet were then compared with the growth and development of rats given a complete and balanced diet, specifically formulated to provide optimum growth. The results of the optimum balanced diet, in terms of growth and development, were assigned a value of 100. A diet restricted to cooked eggs provided enough nutrition to achieve results measured at 78/100. So while eggs provided many of the rats' nutritional needs, they did not allow them to achieve optimal health, or to reach their genetic potential, as defined by the results of the balanced diet.

This is actually an excellent score for a diet consisting of only one food; their score of 78 on a nutritional index meant that these rats were better off than most North Americans today. In terms of the nutritional index, whole milk, with Vitamin D added, achieved a 63 ; enriched white bread managed a 57, cooked potatoes a 48, Canned tuna was 44, polished rice was a mere 29 and *skimmed* milk with vitamins D and A added scraped in at 12 – barely food! Skimmed milk is what so many people are encouraged to feed their children, and yet the rats surviving on skimmed milk barely made it through each day. Gurr's sole nutrient study demonstrated that the lower the fat content of a food, the lower its nutritional index, and the further from optimal health the rats that survived on it.

Fat free = nutrition free

When fat is removed from food there is a real risk that the assimilation of other essential nutrients will be inhibited. It is known that the absorption of calcium, vitamins A, D, E, K, and all the B vitamins is compromised. And when fat is removed from food so are all the micronutrients about which less is known, such as the tocotrienols, sterols, carotenoids and tocopherols, squalene and chlorophyll. These are antioxidants and precursors to cholesterol. Michael Gurr's single food study is an extreme laboratory study, and was carried out only on rats, but it demonstrates definitively that fats offer critical benefits. The health-enhancing properties of fat must be considered before we start arbitrarily eliminating it from nature's food sources and from all our diets, especially those of our children. When fat is taken out of dairy products vitamin A is also removed. Vitamin A is needed for vision and to help our cells with differentiation (replication and maintenance of health) and immunity. Clearly; the less fat in a food, the less vitamin A is available to aid immunity and eye health.

Vitamin D has received so much promotion over the last year for its role in bone development. Supplements fly off the shelf with this kind of good press, yet people are not being encouraged to eat *natural* sources of vitamin D such as lard and full-fat dairy products. Fat-reduced dairy is fortified with synthetic vitamin D after the natural source has been flushed out of the food. Dr. Barbara Sloan notes in her consumer report on fat consumption that health issues around eyes and vision are now a matter of serious concern in North America. Removing the fat from foods decreases intake of the antioxidant vitamin E, leaving cells more susceptible to oxidative damage. Phospholipids, the fats that help build cell membranes, are also at risk of being removed with de-fatting. A diet without phospholipids also offers less protection against ulceration of the stomach and the intestinal lining. Conjugated linoleic acid (CLA, covered in detail in the 'Tango with Butter' chapter) is a fatty acid that has been proven to be beneficial to fat metabolisation. Imagine; a component in fat that ensures fat can be metabolised. Mother Nature really does know what she is doing! CLA also influences growth, helps to metabolise cholesterol, and like vitamin E, functions as an antioxidant. CLA is now a popular trimming supplement and is used more and more as a supplement in animal feed to keep animals leaner.

And one of the most vital roles of fats is their anti-microbial property, which is to say that fats help us to maintain a healthy intestinal flora.

Given all the healthful properties of fat, we have ask why the public is still demanding that fat be removed from products; it's a very important question. As Mrs. X learned, there is no danger to our health, or the health of our children, if we embrace a balanced and moderate diet. My daughter Lucy is now 5 years old and a "big senior" at school (senior kindergarten, that is). She is a whopping 38 pounds, 3½ feet tall, and tremendously enjoys butter and whole grain artisan bread daily. Mayonnaise, cream, *crème fraîche*, Camembert, chocolate eggs, butter, and the Italian pudding *zambonione* made with eggs, cream and sugar are standard fare in our home. Coconut cream pie is my favourite dessert – made with fresh organic ingredients.

Fat is essential for satiety, for the balancing of food cravings, and for the flavour, odour, colour, texture, and palatability of foods. Many predict that fat will be the next newly discovered saviour of our health, the next "functional food" to enjoy celebrity status. Just as Linus Pauling made vitamin C the essential supplement for the common cold, Udo Erasmus in the 1990s brought to light the 'good fat' status of omega 3 and omega 6. And soon the notion that we should strive for a balance of all fats will, quite rightly, be in vogue. Fats have been lumped together and collectively denigrated long enough. Now, with North Americans facing a pandemic of obesity, perhaps it is time to finally approach nutrition with balance and common sense, rather than embrace one arbitrary food fad fanaticism after another. All fats are good and necessary – all natural fats, at least. Fat is not going to kill you, give you heart disease, or make *you* fat. Learn how to use fat properly and effectively and your metabolism will rev up; you'll be more balanced in your thoughts and mood, free of cravings and nutritionally satisfied, and better able to repair the ongoing damage that occurs at the cellular level.

Milk

100 years ago cows produced 400-500 lbs. of milk per year on average. In 2001 they produced 20,000-30,000!

The critical ratio for 0mega-3:Omega-6 utilization is 4:1

Breeding entails a selection for hyperpituitary cows which creates lactating hormone but also growth

Hormones are stored in the water fraction of milk

Fermented dairy makes lactose more digestible. (yogurt, Kefir)

Cultured buttermilk is:
- Low in the difficult to digest casein protein
- High in lactic acid

FAT that is removed also takes
- Steric acid (18 carbons)
- Omega-6
- Chromium
- CLA

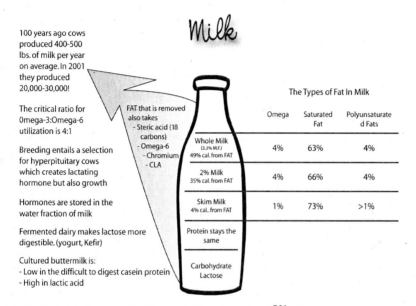

	Omega	Saturated Fat	Polyunsaturated Fats
The Types of Fat In Milk			
Whole Milk (3.3% M.F.) 49% cal. from FAT	4%	63%	4%
2% Milk 35% cal. from FAT	4%	66%	4%
Skim Milk 4% cal.. from FAT	1%	73%	>1%

Protein stays the same

Carbohydrate Lactose

To find the % of calories from fat, use the following equation:

1.8 oz. glass of 2% milk has:
= 6 grams of fat (on the label) per 150 total calories
= 6 grams of fat x 9 calories/gram per 150 total calories
= 54 calories of fat per 150 total calories

= 35% calories from fat!!

CHAPTER 10

OXIDATION FRUSTRATION: THE BAD SIDE OF GOOD OILS

Oxidation: how it works...

Oxidation is a process that is taking place constantly all around us. The rust (iron *oxide*) in a cast iron frying pan, the flame on the stove that's heating the frying pan, the stale sherry-like flavour of a bottle of wine that's been left uncorked; these are all the results of different forms of oxidation. In a very small nutshell, oxidation involves the transfer of electrons, generally in the presence of oxygen, from molecules that lose them to molecules that capture them.

There are two sorts of oxidation that involve dietary fats and oils. The first is a necessary process by which fat is converted by the body into sugars that are then used for energy. This is a complex process of many stages, quite natural and, as I said, necessary. The other form of oxidation involves the breaking down of fatty acids upon contact with, for example, oxygen, metals or salts; this reaction is equally natural, but altogether *unhealthy*. When it takes place in oil in your kitchen, in a badly managed store, or during processing, it renders it increasingly unhealthy, and gives it a particular smell and taste that most of us are familiar with, and instinctively find unpleasant. When it takes place in fatty acids within your body – possibly fatty acids already rendered unstable by the oxidation they've undergone on the shelf next to your stove – the process of oxidation takes the form of an uncontrolled and very much unwanted chain reaction, which involves and damages the molecules of your body's cells. Anti-oxidants shut down this chain reaction, but they are used up in the process, and so your body needs a steady supply – especially if your diet includes too much vegetable oil.

Oxidation is one of the most important factors determining the healthfulness of oils, and yet it is something about which most people, including health practitioners, have little or no knowledge. The oxidation of unsaturated fatty acids is one of the most fundamental reactions in lipid chemistry. When unsaturated oils are exposed to air or excessive heat, to metals, salts or ultraviolet light, complex compounds form which cause rancidity. This reaction will lower the quality of any food in which oils are present. The free radicals (highly reactive molecules with an unbalanced electron count in their outer shells) that result from oxidized lipids cause tissue damage, and this process ultimately plays a part in degenerative diseases such as arthritis, heart disease and many forms of cancer.

It is essential to protect the integrity of unsaturated oils, and from what I have seen in our supermarkets and in the homes of clients, very few people understand this, or give much thought at all to the care of the oils they are eventually going to eat. Expensive, supposedly healthy oils that have not been well cared for are quite likely anything but healthy, and processing fragile unsaturated oils into foods in a way that exposes them to heat and pressure will almost certainly render them harmful. Lipid oxidation is a true frustration.

Why oxidation happens

The oxidation that can take place during the processing of oils will be accelerated by the presence of trace metals such as iron, copper, and zinc, as well as by salt. Careless processing that does not limit the exposure to light, excessive heat and air will also produce substantial levels of oxidation. Fats that are improperly handled during processing usually end up with an off colour and a rancid flavour and odour. This then leads to further processing, such as deodorization and bleaching, to mask these problems. When oils are burnt during stove top cooking, this will cause oxidation as well. Heat, ultraviolet and visible light, and bacteria and moulds that produce lipolytic enzymes (enzymes that break down fat) also catalyse and speed up any oxidation of polyunsaturated oils. The less saturated an oil, the more susceptible it is to oxidation. So the new 'heart-healthy' oils – soybean, safflower, sunflower, and corn oil – carry the greatest risk of uncontrolled oxidation. Canola and olive oils, and oils made from hybrids of safflower and sunflower with higher omega 9 content, oxidise less. And of course the oils least at risk of premature oxidation are the ones that we have been warned not to eat – palm oil, coconut oil, butter and tallow.

Canola, safflower, sunflower, corn and soybean oils have long been the favourites of nutrition-conscience people, because they are highly polyunsaturated. The polyunsaturated content of these oils ranges from 22% in canola to 78% in safflower oil. But being polyunsaturated does not automatically make an oil healthy. We know that oxidized dietary lipids have a direct effect on human health, as significant contributing factors in many chronic diseases and disorders. The uncritical promotion of polyunsaturated fats by governments and medical authorities, and their wholesale addition to processed foods, completely ignore the crucial importance of oil stability; and as a result, they compromise our health. Oxidised polyunsaturated and monounsaturated oils represent a hazard, and require your body to tap into its anti-oxidant stores, and dietary supplies of anti-oxidants, in order to neutralize any oxidation that may have occurred. A diet that is over-dependent on polyunsaturated fats runs the risk of fomenting a free radical riot inside the body, which in turn can easily exhaust the reinforcements of anti-oxidants from vitamin E, beta carotene, zinc, selenium, vitamin C and glutathione that your body holds in reserve to keep the peace. The result can be an inner landscape of broken windows and burnt-out cars.

As well as destroying essential fatty acids and using up anti-oxidants, oxidation produces toxic compounds and oxidized polymers. Polymers arise through the formation of either carbon-to-carbon bonds or oxygen bridges between fat molecules. This is most likely to occur during the most common commercial methods of processing or heating. When too many polymers are present in an oil there is a marked increase in viscosity, and the polymers will be poorly absorbed from the intestinal tract. Even a simple process such as crushing seeds or nuts for baking in a cake at home can cause metals and proteins to dissociate, and metals such as iron, with their many free electrons, may bind to any free fatty acid and catalyse lipid oxidation.

Water can also accelerate oxidation as well, by making dissolved metals more available for reaction, and by allowing greater, more immediate contact between these dissolved metals and the fats and oils present in food. Refrigeration and vacuum packaging of food prevent oxidation by controlling water activity. Even in a food like milk, which is dense in fatty acids, the oxidation rate of phospholipids is dependent on whether the fatty parts are suspended in water or fat. For example, homogenized milk has higher oxidative stability than non-homogenized milk because of the resurfacing of the fat with the protein casein, which provides a protective layer and prevents contact with water.

In meat and poultry, oxidation occurs initially in the phospholipids of cellular and subcellular membranes which are in close proximity to the metal catalyst iron. Lipid oxidation is accelerated when meat's structure is disrupted through simple preparations such as tenderizing, grinding, heating or chopping. These expose the phospholipids to oxygen, enzymes and heme pigments (our blood is red because of the iron in these pigments), which can all cause oxidation.

The fatty acid ratios of meats also influence the rate of oxidation. Chicken and turkey meats are more susceptible to oxidation than beef is, because of their higher polyunsaturated phospholipid content. And the dark meat of poultry oxidises even faster, because it has a high polyunsaturated content, as well as more of the catalyst iron than is found in white meat. In cured meats sodium nitrite is used as an inhibitor of lipid oxidation, and is the source of its red colour. Grandma Doolittle used natural antioxidants found in rosemary extracts to extend the life of meat. Rosemary extracts contain potent antioxidants and are effective in stabilizing cooked pork, beef, chicken and turkey. Fish is also subject to lipid oxidation. Synthetic antioxidants such as BHT and BHA are often added to fish during processing, and fish themselves have high levels of tocopherols and flavonoids, which are natural antioxidants. In processing plants and at sea, the measures used to prevent rancidity include limiting exposure to air and vacuum sealing products.

In short; all the delicate food oils that we consume, and especially the newer vegetable oils that have increased so dramatically in our diets since the turn of the last century, need to be processed and handled with care in order to avoid unnecessary lipid oxidation and the associated health risks. We now find polyunsaturated oil in salad dressings, in dips like hummus or baba ganoush, in prepared coleslaws and salads, in "healthy" versions of chips, crackers, dried breads, corn chips and tortillas, in fresh breads, flat breads, frozen foods, frozen prepared meals, baby foods, cold cereals, cookies, pastries, energy bars, and protein bars… and *all* these foods expose us to harm because of the degradation of the unstable oils they contain. This is the oxidation frustration that comes with polyunsaturated fats.

All foods with fats in them, even grains and cereals, require precautions to minimize oxidation. Store grains in the fridge or freezer if you can. Keep polyunsaturated oils in opaque bottles at a constant temperature, and keep the lids on — oils should always be stored sealed tight. Don't leave the butter on the counter; keep it in the fridge. If you want soft butter, cut off just what you need for the day. We intuitively know what oxidation is; our bodies have good reason to recoil from the smell and taste of food that's so bad for us. The process of oxidation is a very important factor determining not just how an oil tastes, but also its nutritional quality, bioavailability and even its potential toxicity – in the sense of leading to the development of disease.

Oxidation and fried foods

In 1984, fast food restaurants became the targets of government and media criticism for using saturated fat to fry their foods, and so running foul of the official consensus that all saturated fat, no matter the circumstances in which it is used, is deadly. At the same time, vegetarian groups were rallying against the evils of hidden animal fats in deep fried foods. It wasn't long before deep fryers everywhere were refilled with predominately unsaturated oils in various degrees of hydrogenation, or with genetically engineered oils. Tallow, until then the most common animal fat in fryers, was history. Canola, soybean and 'mixed vegetable' oils flooded into restaurant fryers, and so into customers, all across North America.

There is no such thing as 'healthy frying'. But it tastes good! And there's no reason why fried food shouldn't be eaten in moderation, as part of a diet that's also rich in free radical scavenging foods. And the unhealthiest thing about fried food is the free radical damage that high heat inflicts on the unsaturated fatty acids found in safflower, sunflower, soybean, corn, and mixed vegetable oil blends. When saturated fats (butter, coconut, and to a lesser extent lard and tallow) are used in frying, the oil suffers less oxidative damage. When we eat less-damaged fats, we help preserve the body's supply of anti-oxidants, since there are fewer oxidized molecules to be eliminated. Deep-fried foods were originally regarded as taboo only because they absorb more fat and calories than other forms of cooking, regardless of the saturation point of the oil used. Funnily enough, we we now know that short chain *saturated* fats have a lower absorption rate and caloric concentration than longer chain *unsaturated* fats.

Using unsaturated oil for frying does not make fried foods healthier! It is not saturation that makes a fried oil healthy or unhealthy, but the degree to which the fat will break down to create free radicals and trans isomers. The toxicity of heated oils – the extent to which heat-damaged oils will potentially interfere with the biochemical reactions that keep cells healthy – varies from one type of fat to the next. This is why it's important to choose the most stable oils for frying. The amount of heated oil in a food and the frequency of exposure affect the way in which toxic molecules interact with the molecules of our bodies. How well we detoxify the toxic by-products of frying (dimmers, cross-linked fatty acid chains, linked triglycerides, bond-shifted fatty acids, and polymers) will depend largely on the quality of our whole diet and the health of our bodies' systems.

Lard can be more unsaturated than saturated, depending on the diet of the pig. And lard is predominately home rendered, which also results in a varying mixture of different sorts of fat. The harder the lard the better suited it is for high heat cooking; lard that is liquid at room temperature should be treated and used as an unsaturated fat. Refined trans configuration fats and fully saturated fats with low essential fatty acids actually suffer the least oxidative damage when fried, and pass the least damage on to us. Olive, safflower, sunflower and soybean oils, on the other hand, ultimately *increase* the risk of coronary heart disease, arthritis, and elevated cholesterol levels when fried – because they are not stable, and because they increase the inflammatory response. Remember; if you choose to eat fried food, it is not for the health benefits, but for the flavour.

To summarise: never, ever fry with flaxseed oil or hemp seed oil. In fact, don't cook with them at all. Avoid frying or high heat cooking with sunflower, soybean, safflower, and corn oils, as they are all high in omega 6 and deteriorate rapidly. High oleic sunflower and safflower oils are made from genetically modified versions of these plants, and have exchanged omega 6 concentration for omega 9 concentration. They can be used for frying and are now more widely available than just a few years ago. Canola and olive oils have roughly equal amounts of omega 9 and omega 6 and will therefore be somewhat stable during stove top frying, but you might want to blend them with the saturated fat in a tablespoon of butter. The shorter the frying time, the less damage is incurred by oil and the food you're frying in it. The best oils for frying are stable ones such as butter, cocoa butter, palm, palm kernel, and coconut oil. The make-up of lard varies depending on the method of rendering and the diet of the swine, but for the most part lard is stable enough for stove top frying.

CHAPTER 11
OMEGA 6: OMEGA 3 RATIOS, A MODERN DILEMMA

"With respect to the contemporary diet, the n-6:n-3 fatty acid ratio has changed significantly...a typical Western diet [is] characterized by foods high in refined carbohydrates, trans fatty acids, and vegetable oils high in Omega 6...A growing number of scientists believe the present level of n-6:n-3 ratio is involved in the development of many chronic diseases." [3]

"The lack of differentiation between the essential polyunsaturated fatty acids Omega 6 and Omega 3 we are today medicating away disease that is very much connected to our imbalanced ratios of omega 6 and omega 3 fatty acids." [4]

"Cancer is among the main causes of mortality worldwide, and is the second leading cause of death in Canada and the United States. ...by all estimates 30% of cancer risk is associated with diet." [5]

Omega 6- less is more

Most consumers haven't yet managed to school themselves in the intricacies of the symbiotic relationship between the two essential fatty acids, omega 6 and omega 3. Taking their cues from the pronouncements of media and government, people still tend to focus haphazardly on one beneficial trait of a particular nutrient, as we are now doing with omega 6, assuming that its one good quality (that it is a polyunsaturated fatty acid) represents the sum of its effects on our metabolism and health. Well, as you probably know by now; that is not how these things work. Omega 6, when eaten to excess and out of proportion to other essential fatty acids, has a negative side, and it is having an enormously negative effect on our health – more than anyone wants to admit just yet. For example; in my own practise I have seen almost unbelievable results undoing obesity with proper management of fats and oils, including adjustments to omega 6 ratios. Just because some omega 6 is good for us doesn't mean that a lot of it is better, or even harmless.

Omega 6 is currently ubiquitous in our diets; and our lack of awareness regarding its essential functions, and the importance of eating enough but not too much, has us consuming it without caution. The sooner you can decrease your reliance on omega 6 fats and increase the amount of omega 3 you consume, the sooner your body's systems will begin to recover from the damage caused by overdosing on omega 6, as almost all of have been doing over the last several decades. It is time to get to work on creating the paradigm shift that redefines omega 6 fats, in the quantities we consume them today, as harmful. We have to understand that the term 'polyunsaturated' is not a synonym for 'healthy'.

It seems like omega 6 and omega 3 fats have been in the spotlight continuously for the past two decades, as the stars of a new and exciting breakthrough in nutritional understanding. But Rudolf Virchow was studying their essential roles as far back as the 1840s. Despite this long history, until very recently linoleic and linolenic acids – omega 6 and 3 fatty acids – were so poorly understood that they were dealt with as if they were one and the same substance. A.J. Vergrossen's 1975 book *The Role of Fats In Human Nutrition,* the definitive collection on fats at the time, referred throughout to the omega fatty acids as only omega 6/ linoleic acid. Linolenic acid, the omega 3 essential fatty acid, was considered to be too similar, and present in concentrations too low, to be significant. As recently as the 1980s university nutrition curricula largely neglected the importance of omega 3.

The inherently synergistic relationship between these two nutrients was misunderstood for a long time. This has had serious consequences, as an imbalance of these fats will show up in the constitution of our tissues. The fats we eat are built into our cells, which receive eicosanoids (long chain hormone-like inflammatory and anti/inflammatory mediators) to promote either inflammatory or non-inflammatory response. The type of eicosanoid secretion is influenced by its omega 6 or omega 3 precursors. Omega 6 eicosanoids, which promote inflammatory response, are more hardy and aggressive than omega 3 eicosanoids. Excessive omega 6 eicosanoids in our systems can lead to a state of chronic disease if they are not moderated by sufficient competing omega 3 eicosanoids. So again, a little omega 6 is good, too much is just plain bad!

For decades research in this area was slowed down by the assumption that the essential fatty acids were so similar that they couldn't have different physiological affects. This delayed our understanding of the way that omega 3 and 6 are not simply different nutrients, but complimentary ones; their symbiotic relationship, if it is to function properly, requires a balance between the opposing effects they initiate. We now know that maintaining an appropriate omega 6-omega 3 ratio is fundamental to good health. And yet, while manufactured food products have been modified to increase our intake of polyunsaturated oils, the focus is squarely on omega 6 rich oils. Omega 3 has conveniently been ignored. And 'conveniently' is just the right word; omega 3 has routinely been processed out of products precisely because its instability, as a highly unsaturated fat, inconveniently shortens their shelf life.

Ensuring the right balance of omega 6 to omega 3 in our diets is essential for optimum health. And yet products that are high in omega 6 polyunsaturated fat continue to flood the aisles of supermarkets, while fish products and flax seeds and oils, all rich in omega 3, have shown no increase in consumption – have perhaps even shown a decrease. And while consumers have been only too aware of the conditions and diseases caused by this imbalance, they have *not* been made aware of the role that it plays. And as a result the imbalance has worsened from one generation to the next. The polyunsaturated fats rich in omega 6, as a single undifferentiated category, have continued to be promoted as the royal road to health, to be substituted at every opportunity for the saturated fats in butter, lard, and beef fat. This is behaviour without any basis in nutritional reality.

Oils rich in omega 6 affect our bodies' systems as soon as we begin to eat them. Their effects grow and compound as we mature and continue to eat these oils. The affects of omega 6 increase cumulatively over time, as they are literally built into our cells and systems.

Essential fatty acids are converted into tissue structures and also mediate tissue signalling, setting the body up to receive signals for inflammatory or anti-inflammatory responses. Both omega 6 and omega 3 are construction materials, continuously formed and reformed by our bodies – partly in proportion to their concentrations in our diets, and partly according to their ability to compete for the vitamin co-factors necessary for these transformations. In other words, fatty acids are constantly in flux, and in competition for co-factors that help them perform their prescribed roles within the body. The most abundant fatty acid in the diet will have the greatest affect on biological reactions, and so the relative proportion of the different fatty acids in our diets will strongly influence our health. Excessive vegetable oil in one meal or snack can affect inflammatory pathways for long periods of time, until the stimulating fat is removed from the system. You could have an extended *anti-inflammatory* response if you are prone to overeating fatty fish, drinking flaxseed oil or eating flax seeds, but for most people the pro-inflammatory pathway is the one that is overstimulated, due to the excessive concentration of omega 6 oils and omega 6 rich processed foods in our diets.

When good fats behave badly

"The epidemic of cardiovascular disease among Americans (along with its associated disorder, obesity) comes from a public health environment that has failed to educate people adequately about when food gives benefits or harm. ...Imbalances in the intake and expenditure of energy and in the intakes of omega 3, omega 6 EFA are causing a tragic epidemic of cardiovascular deaths among Americans. These two readily prevented imbalances cause vascular damage...Diseases caused by such imprudence can be prevented with better lifelong advice to the public about foods and lipid metabolism. Current treatments that fail to correct the dietary imbalances that cause disease leave patients vulnerable to continued lifelong dependence on expensive mediations and treatments."[6]

Here is the real dilemma with respect to essential fatty acid intake; the average diet in North America is chronically low in omega 3, and excessively high in omega 6 and polyunsaturated trans-fatty acids. As mentioned in the discussion of food consumption patterns, our intake of vegetable oils rich in both omega 6 and omega 9 has increased by close to 400% since the turn of the last century. Omega 6 competes directly with omega 3 for the same enzymes and vitamin co-factors necessary to make omega 3 into the highly unsaturated fatty acids that are found *pre-formed* in fish. The end products of the converted omega oils are predominately used in the brain, sex glands, and nervous system. The issue is not simply that we consume insufficient omega 3: competition for enzymes and co-factors from omega 6 makes the omega 3 deficit even greater. Omega 6 should convert into the highly unsaturated fatty acid derivatives at a rate comparable to omega 3's conversion into its version of superunsaturated fatty acids. However, because of the long-standing imbalance of these oils in the diet, the dominant fat, omega 6, converts into pro-inflammatory stimuli like a rabbit runs, while omega 3 converts into anti-inflammatory stimuli like a tortoise crawls.

To compound the problem; we simply don't eat omega 3 in significant concentrations any more. We don't eat enough fish, flaxseed, hemp, pumpkin oil, walnut, eyeballs, blubber, or insects. There is a constant, unremitting oversupply of omega 6, and as a result our bodies keep producing the inflammatory and immune-suppressing responses that fuel arthritis, allergies, asthma, cancer, PMS, weight gain, cardiovascular disease, diverse auto-immune problems, and cardiac arrhythmia, to name a few particularly modern disorders.

On average, North Americans currently consume about 20 times as much omega 6 as omega 3. The *recommended* ratio is between three and four parts omega 6 to one part omega 3; this ratio would allow optimum conversion of both fats into the very important super-unsaturated fatty acids. But of the four oils that predominate in North American diets, corn oil has 46 times as much omega 6 as omega three, and cotton seed, safflower and sunflower oils have *more than 250 times as much*. See how far we have moved away from nutritional and biological balance! The current omega 6 recommendations do not reflect science or common sense. And many people are unable to recover from the metabolic diseases that result, because their diet imposes a gross nutritional imbalance that continually feeds the problem. Yet we are still not being encouraged to abandon our collective mania for polyunsaturated oils. This is the elephant in the committee room of the food policy administrators. We need to stop eating safflower, sunflower, soybean, corn, and to a lesser extent canola oils, and all foods made with them. Do not seek them out! Avoid them! Do not replace your vital saturated fats with these oils!

Nutrition information produced for popular consumption has routinely shown the same pattern; over-simplified interpretations of a science still in progress have been used as the basis for sweeping warnings and recommendations. Then it has taken years to change or undo policy and propaganda that should never have seen the light of day in the first place. The about-turns over refined carbohydrates, hydrogenation and trans fatty acids represent just three examples in which nutritional wisdom had to be abandoned and rewritten, and then re-communicated to consumers in the form of a new set of rules closer to the real truth.

When it came to learning about trans fatty acids, consumers made a lot of headway on their own, and educated themselves before they put pressure on government and industry. We can do the same with omega 6 fatty acids – and it is time we started. While the issue remains below the radar of media and policy-makers, a few researchers (and only a few, so far) have written in lay terms on this subject; further reading will help solidify your understanding, and hopefully make clear the importance of acting quickly.

Mary Enig is a lipid biochemist who has teamed up with the writer Sally Fallon to write a remarkably concise essay, available on the Internet, called *The Oiling of America*. The essay presents a political hypothesis for the dominance of polyunsaturated oil since the 1950s, as well as covering the basics of polyunsaturated biochemistry. There is also an excellent textbook for the more advanced reader by renowned biologist and writer Michael Gurr; *Lipids in Nutrition: a Health Reappraisal*. Once you start to explore this literature other resources will come your way. My prediction is that the domination of the consumer's nutritional imagination by omega6/polyunsaturated fats will be overcome in the next four or five years.

What follows is the nitty-gritty on how these wonderful 'good fats' get converted into fatty acids that are the same as those found in fish. It is important to understand that the conversion will work efficiently only to the extent that a diet is balanced in all the other nutrients that support the conversions, and that the precursor fats will not be converted if there is any fundamental impediment in the system. Most of us have nutritionally unbalanced diets, so conversion rates can be very, very low. This is especially critical for pregnant and nursing mothers, because their nutritional needs are so great, and for children and the elderly, who tend to have more restricted diets, involving less food and less variety. The progression of conversions is dependent, at different points, on the minerals iron, zinc and magnesium and the vitamins B6, B3 and C. Along the way conversions can be impeded by: high cholesterol, high blood sugar, high blood-alcohol levels, the presence of trans fatty acids, over-consumption of 'bad oils', as in vegetable oils that are higher in omega 9, consumption of processed and heated oils, illnesses such as diabetes, and (unfortunately) by ageing.

Omega 6/ linoleic acid's first conversion is by delta-6-desaturase (D-6-D) into gamma-linolenic acid (GLA). GLA is found pre-formed in evening primrose oil, borage oil and black current seed oil. These oils are used predominately as 'nutriceuticals' (foods with significant medicinal qualities) to aid common inflammatory complaints, such as pre-menstrual syndrome. GLA then interacts with the enzyme elongase, which transforms it into an even longer fatty acid chain. It is converted into di-hommogamma-linolenic acid (DGLA), which is abundant in mothers' milk. GLA is now available in supplement form, mixed in with other essential fatty acids, because a portion of the population cannot convert linoleic acid to gamma-linolenic acid efficiently.

The delta-6-desaturase enzyme that is responsible for the conversion is said to be the *rate-limiting enzyme* for omega 6 conversion. D-6-D is always present in our system but must be accompanied by adequate cofactors, such as zinc and iron, to work efficiently. So GLA supplements in the form of evening primrose oil, borage oil, or black current seed oil help bypass the deficiency or blocked enzyme, and the system can con-

tinue to initiate the release of prostaglandins that the body needs to mod-
ulate inflammation. DGLA stimulates the release of prostaglandin 1. This
is an anti-inflammatory stimulus. So tissues with a high concentration
of omega 6 would receive the anti-inflammatiory prostaglandin stimulus
initiated during the conversion phase of this fatty acid. It would have
mere seconds to exert an anti-inflammation response on tissues with a
high concentration of omega 6. Then, as the fat continued on its career
through elongation and desaturation each step would stimulate a new inflammatory or anti-inflammatory response. Dihomogamma-linolenic
would then convert to arachidonic acid, which stimulates the release of
prostagladin 2, and thromboxanes, and series 4 leukotrienes, all of which
mediate full-on inflammation at the tissue destination. Although there is
one step in omega 6 metabolism that mediates an anti-inflammatory response, most of the stimulus is pro-inflammatory.

All omega 6 must pass through this conversion. There are four more
conversion steps before the fatty acid is ready for beta-oxidation, which
is the stage at which a fat is ready to be used for the metabolism. Along
the way there is a constant demand for nutrients and co-factors to convert
each intermediate fatty acid into the next stage in the series. Sophisticated blood tests that come to me from executive medical exams indicate
which fatty acids are accumulating in the system. These are good bio-
markers, as they show which stage of the conversion system is the weak-
est and which fatty acids need attention – or which co-factors need to be
supplemented. If someone is suffering from an autoimmune disease related to fatty acid imbalance, such as eczema or fibromyalgia, a fatty acid
profile could be the starting point to correcting the weakness.

Omega 3 fatty acids must go through four conversions, from their
original composition as dietary linolenic fatty acid, before they can release the opposing set of anti-inflammatory eicosanoids. Omega 3 is ingested as alpha-linolenic acid. It must first compete with omega 6 for
delta 6 desaturase (D-6-D) enzymes to convert into stearidonic acid.
(18:4w3) If it makes it this far, it then goes on to convert into eicosate-
traenoic acid (ETA: 20:4w3). At this point the omega 3 derivatives have
not yet had an opportunity to exert their anti-inflammatory properties.
The next conversion is to eicosapentaenoic acid (EPA; 20:5w3) but in
order for this to happen, the ETA has to compete for the delta 5 desat-

urase enzyme. If it makes it to this stage, the EPA stimulates the release of the anti-inflammatory Prostaglandins PGE1, PGH3, PGI3, and thromboxane A3, as well as leukotrienes series 5.

This is a difficult journey for omega 3. I liken it to baby turtles racing to make the treacherous journey from their nests to the waters edge before they are picked off by predators. And our bodies still have to perform four more successful conversions before DHA, the essential fatty acid in childhood development, brain, eye, nerve, and gene expression, is created. The omega 6 conversion is far more aggressive, *as well as being able to secure a greater proportion of vitamin co-factors because omega 6 is so abundant in the diet.* All the omega 6-related systems are on high alert, and constantly exercising their tissue stimulation functions. So even as the omega 3 fatty acids release anti-inflammatory response signals, the omega 6 are getting their contrary signals out at a much faster rate, virtually suppressing the function of omega 3 fatty acid derivatives.

In dietary terms, it adds up to this; only a tiny proportion of the omega 3 we ingest is successfully converted – the estimated rate is about 3.8% for women, and 1% for men. And most of our natural sources of omega 3 fatty acids also contain omega 6, which is already too abundant in our diet. In this extreme situation, the only way to re-balance our internal ratios of omega 6 and 3 is to increase our intake of omega 3-rich foods, while *decreasing* omega 6 intake, and perhaps even taking additional omega 3 supplements until an optimum balance is realized.

Rebalancing fatty acid ratios: making 'good fats' better

Dr. Udo Erasmus, acclaimed omega fats expert and author of *Fats that Heal, Fats that Kill*, advises supplementing with flaxseed oil for three to six months in order to drag the balance of fats back to a healthy ratio. His recommendation is one tablespoon for every 100 pounds of lean body mass, daily for three months. (Lean body mass is your weight without the fat). At the end of this period, a diet containing a balanced proportion of all fats should be followed. Alternatively, an imbalance can be corrected over the course of a few months by consuming a few 8.5 oz bottles of good quality flaxseed oil. *Continued supplementation with omega 3 is not recommended.* Once re-balance has been achieved, stop supplementing! Remember the omega 3s are highly unsaturated oils and they oxidise rapidly. Excess oxidation will undo the health benefits of the oil. Constant supplementation with fish oils is one of the most widespread errors I see in my practice. This is a good example of the critical importance of keeping a food log; it will ensure that you don't overdo a good thing with the fish oil.

After the saturation point has been reached with respect to omega 3, it is critical to stick to dietary habits that provide roughly four parts omega 6 to one part omega 3. A successfully balanced diet would involve minimising the intake of all the common vegetable based oils. If such a dietary regimen seems too daunting a task, then consider achieving a healthier internal balance of oils (eventually!) by simply increasing your consumption of food sources rich in omega 3, and decreasing your consumption of omega 6.

To help re-establish omega balance, eat plenty of these foods;
- Flaxseeds, and Flaxseed oil
- Salba (chia)
- Fish for its pre-formed DHA and EPA

The other nuts and seeds rich in omega 3 also have high concentrations of omega 6; to remedy an omega imbalance it is probably best to avoid nuts and seeds for two months.

DHA and EPA: the fish fats and omega 3 derivatives

The 'fish fats' are eicosapentanoic acid, abbreviated as EPA or 20:5w3, and docosahexaenoic acid - DHA or 22:6w3. Omega 3 and omega 6 provide the precursor nutrients for making these super-polyunsaturated fatty acids, otherwise known as highly unsaturated fatty acids (HUFA). DHA and EPA have garnered much of the attention once focused on the original 'good fats'. These long chain fatty acids are found predominantly in fatty fish and fish oil supplements. Nuts and seeds such as hemp, pumpkin, flax, walnut and soy contain only omega 3 linolenic acid, not the pre-formed DHA. It is impossible to get these fats if you are a vegetarian! Sardines, salmon, mackerel, trout, and eel have the highest concentration of EPA and DHA, while all other fish contain lesser amounts. About a quarter of the fatty acid profile of shellfish is EPA and DHA, but these are lean creatures — only about 2% fat by weight, so it follows that their fatty acid content will also be very low. Raw fish such as sushi and sashimi has the best quality of these longer chain fatty acids. Otherwise, fish oils are most plentiful in fish that has been boiled, as this minimises the breakdown of the essential fats compared to other cooking methods. The skin and the underbelly are the richest sources of omega fats, which are also found in abundance behind the gills and around the fins; so eating *whole* fish, with the *skin on*, is the healthiest way to go. Fillets just aren't the same, but they will do until your pallet is conditioned to more flavourful fatty textures and tastes.

EPA and DHA are derivatives of omega 3, and are most needed in the most active locations in the human body; in nerve synapses throughout the body and especially within the brain, sex organs, retina, adrenal glands and inner ear. If you want to get the kids to hear you the first time, make sure they eat fish!

Dr. Sheila Innes from the University of British Columbia has done extensive research on DHA intake and needs. Her research shows a direct linear relationship between DHA intake and blood profiles. If you are eating the fish, these important fatty acids are making it to your tissues. But if you depend on plant sources to supplement your DHA needs, you can't be as confident that bioavailable DHA will result.

A recommended daily DHA/EPA intake is not yet established, but the Dietetic Association have decided not to wait for regulation, and are recommending an intake of 200-400 mg per day. The average Canadian intake is 130 mg per day, with 42% of the population eating below 20 mg per day. (Inuit eat, on average, 2200 mg of DHA and EPA per day!) So if you eat a typical Canadian diet, you only need to add two more servings of fish per week to meet your need for these fatty acids.

I believe that North Americans' overconsumption of omega 6 fatty acids represents one of the most damaging aspects of our chronically unbalanced diets. Like the others – such as our reliance on processed food stripped of all its nutrition in factories the size of auto assembly plants, and our incredible consumption of sugar and corn syrup – it is a direct consequence of our having let 'experts', and the commercial interests of the food industry, override the intuitive understanding of nutrition that is inherent in most traditional diets. And the relationship between over-consumption of omega 6 laden vegetable oils and the diseases that define ill-health in the modern age, from allergies and arthritis to diabetes and obesity to cancer and heart disease, is becoming clearer all the time.

3. S. Gebauer et al. 2005. Dietary n-6:n-3 Fatty Acid Ratio and Health, in Oi-Ming Lai and Casimir C. Akoh eds *Healthful Lipids* AOCS Publishing, pg 228.
4. William E.M. Lands Essential Fatty Acid Metabolism to Self-Healing Agents, in Oi-Ming Lai and Casimir C. Akoh eds *Healthful Lipids* AOCS Publishing, pg. 205
5. Breanne Anderson and David W.L. Ma. 2009. Fatty Acids in Membrane Lipids: Role in Disease Causation and Prevention. In Ronald R. Watson ed. *Fatty Acids in Health Promotion and Disease Causation.* ENG Publishing.
6. William E.M. Lands. 2005. Essential Fatty Acid Metabolism to Self-Healing Agents in Oi-Ming Lai and Casimir C. Akoh eds *Healthful Lipids* AOCS Publishing.

CHAPTER 12
OPTIMISING DHA AND EPA

"CANADIAN CHILDREN HAVE THE 'LOWEST' LEVELS
OF DHA IN THE DEVELOPED WORLD!" [7]

DHA and children's health

Recent research by Dr. Shelia Innes shows that maternal DHA deficiency affects the embryonic maturation of neurons, and results in lowered DHA concentrations in mother's milk. DHA is important for the *neurogenesis* (the development of nerves, especially in the brain) that occurs in human foetuses between 3 and 6 months of gestation. The foetus needs to accumulate about 70 mg per day of DHA in the last trimester, but about 40% of pregnant women consume less than 70 mg per day, and the figure is the same for lactating women. If it isn't in a mother's blood during gestation, or in her milk during infancy, then her child is starting life already deficient in a nutrient crucially important for brain development. Many woman who have had children know that fish is one of the foods that can produce a strong aversion during pregnancy; so this would be a good time to rely on supplementation, either with cod liver oil or fish oil capsules. If plugging your nose while you eat it doesn't let you get the fish down, revert to supplementation.

DHA deficiency has an impact on health, particularly on the health of children. And in children, health and development can never be separated; the consequences of poor childhood health and poor childhood nutrition can last a lifetime, though the primary symptoms that result from poor nutrition can be ameliorated with improved diet. In the case of children born in a state of DHA and/or EPA deficiency, low concentration can have consequences for behaviour and intelligence, and improved development during childhood depends on an increased intake of these nutrients. *Children's diets should provide them with at least 200 mg per day of DHA.* This is difficult to achieve without eating fatty fish and/or taking supplements.

Growing awareness concerning the vital need for DHA, given our low fish consumption, has spawned an industry providing foods fortified with DHA. The new technique of *microencapsulating* DHA and EPA protects them against oxidation during processing. This has allowed these nutrients to be added to foods that would otherwise not contain them; orange juice with DHA, bread with DHA, and even Danon Yoghurt with DHA. Ultimately these 'DHA fortified foods' are no match for a fish dinner or a spoonful of fish oil. A child will not be able to get all their DHA requirements from fortified foods alone, and these foods should be seen as supplements, not replacements.

There is no way around it; we have to get our children eating real food again. The agreed-upon DHA/EPA requirements for adults can be met by eating three to four four-ounce servings of fish per week. If you are going to miss that target, or an assessment suggests you have been in an omega 6 dominant state for some time, your diet should probably be supplemented with EPA and DHA fish oils. Because these oils are such potent anti-inflammatories, a sufficient intake should result in a lessening of inflammatory-related symptoms. For example, I know when my diet is lacking in fish oils because of the pre-menstrual symptoms I'll experience. If I have no symptoms, which is actually normal, then I know my anti-inflammatory quota is being met, but if I do get a backache I'm reminded to watch my diet and increase my fish intake. Other mild symptoms that respond quickly to improved EPA and DHA status are sore finger joints, asthma, and knee arthritic pain. Deficiencies of EPA and DHA negatively affect mood, behaviour, libido, vision, and energy.

Personal experiences with kids and fish

My experience as a mother has opened my eyes to the demands of childhood nutrition. It's not an easy task feeding kids, and once they start going to school and learning all the foibles and tricks of the other children the challenge can be insurmountable. While I was breast-feeding my daughter, I would take about 1000 mg worth of fish-oil capsules daily.

This was balanced with a diet and supplements rich in anti-oxidants. At the time I was a spokesperson for a flaxseed oil company, and used the spiced-up flax oil regularly. I admit that fish was not a food I relished during parts of my pregnancy, and even during the early stages of Lucy's infancy. During the weeks when my fish intake was low I would top up with as much as 2000mg of supplemental fish oils per day.

I let the demands of my career force me to stop breast-feeding at three months. Initially I was committed to breastfeeding for at least a year; I was a typically overzealous and idealistic new mother. But the middle-of-the-night feedings were killing me when I still had to work at 6 am, and I was exhausted and looking for ways to sort out my commitments. Like most women who stop breastfeeding I took great care in choosing the formula that I had sworn I would never let my child have. I would mix the formula with the water – and then add a half-teaspoon of flaxseed oil to a bottle. The next bottle got a bit of melted coconut oil, and the next after that a dash of cod liver oil. The formulas now on the market are far more advanced than those available to us just a few years ago. DHA is now added to formula, and it wasn't then, nor was lauric acid from coconut oil. I find it astonishing that these essential fatty acids were added to pet foods long before we considered giving them as supplements to our children.

By the time Lucy started to eat solid food she was most attracted to the really fatty underbelly of the fish – the part that was wet and dripping with fat. I'm not sure whether this was a consequence of her fatty formula diet, but she loved that stuff. I discovered this one day when she gobbled some up before I'd had a chance to scrape it into the garbage. The only people I knew of that would eat that part of the fish were Grandma Doolittle and Nona Santilli. I'm still a modern omnivore, eating the fillet and picking at the rest of the fish. Lucy continued to get infusions of oil mixed into her formula with the bottle that she had with her nap until she was two years old. She was about 22 months old before she threw the bottle back at me; she always fussed about her fish oil/formula mix after a neighbour introduced her to apple juice at nap time!

DHA saturation is a good status to maintain. Some research shows that excess DHA intake has a neutral affect on DHA concentrations in your body – in other words, not elevating them beyond what the body needs. The consensus is that the body will not respond to an excess with any adverse or abnormal reaction, but because the oxidation of super-unsaturated fats represents a risk I would use caution and supplement within the recommended ranges. Oxidation is a real threat, and perhaps there are tipping points that we don't yet know about. Just as our current diet typically provides us with too much omega 6, it might be possible to accumulate too much DHA. The Inuit, with their average daily intake of 2200 mg of EPA and DHA in a ratio of 2:1 respectively, are relatively healthy, though they do experience stroke and cerebral haemorrhage at a far higher rate than the Canadian average. (Omega 3 fats are anti-coagulants and thin the blood.) An excess of fish oils seems to affect cellular integrity and blood viscosity, making it difficult to recover from trauma. Again; some is good, too much is not good.

Children's DHA supplements often come in the form of a chewable orange-flavoured capsule. Lucy's assessment of this particular supplement is that it is barely tolerable, but she is proud to be able to take responsibility for supplementing her own nutrition, and right now she will do anything to avoid having to eat fish! Paolo does make a wonderful breaded fish that Lucy loves. Even though the skin is removed and it is cooked at higher than ideal, stove-top temperatures, it is better than no fish at all. Remember that fish chowders and fish cakes are often a delightful surprise for even the fussiest fish eaters. If your child likes tuna, blend it with canned or fresh salmon. Or bake white fish with a cheddar cheese topping. Or just plain bribe them; that has always worked.

Methyl mercury in fish

"There is a great risk of not eating fish to avoid eating the limited mercury in the fish." [8]

The concentration of mercury in fish remains a valid matter for concern. Research shows that every 1 ppm (part per million) of methyl mercury found in human hair corresponds to an average .18 point loss in IQ. However, there is an average 2.1 point increase in IQ with a weekly intake of 340 grams of fish. So it's all about choosing the right fish, lowest in mercury; and a great deal of information is available to help you make the right choices. We can choose to abstain from eating fish because of the methyl mercury risk, or we can again choose moderation and balance, based on an informed assessment of the risks and benefits.

How to maintain a positive omega 3 status

Once supplementation has achieved DHA saturation, return to eating a 4-6 ounce serving of fish at least 3-4 times per week. Use flaxseed oil alternately with olive oil for salads, and add a few nuts, in particular walnuts and flaxseeds, a few times per week into yoghurt and salads. Or eat them with fruit as a snack. The body will start to incorporate the supply of DHA and omega 3 fats right away, and move towards a balanced omega 3 status. Watch out for packaged foods! Hummus, corn chips, specialty crackers, baked goods, bean salads, prepared soups, and salad dressings will all contain omega 6-rich vegetable oils. I suggest that omega 3 eggs be cooked without breaking the yolk, as this will protect the cholesterol and unsaturated fats from oxidation.

Here is an example of a day's food that would be rich in omega 3 fats. Two poached or boiled omega 3 eggs will give you 800 mg of omega 3 fatty acid, along with plenty of vitamin E, zinc, and selenium to neutralize the oxidation of fatty acids, and 180mg of DHA in its pre-formed state. Add a slice of smoked salmon on a small piece of spelt toast and you've got a substantial daily dose of omega 3, without too much omega 6. For lunch use a full tablespoon of flaxseed oil for your tuna fish salad, sprinkle two tablespoons of pumpkin seeds into your salad and have a hemp bar for dessert with a green tea rich in antioxidants. By dinner you're already at home plate as far as omega 3 is concerned; have the steak and potatoes with sour cream and lots of vegetables. Switch your daily habits and try to avoid the rut of eating the same preferred foods; for breakfast, have yoghurt with a mixture of walnuts, flax, pumpkin and hemp one day, and eggs the next.

I feel that topping up on anti-oxidants with a fish oil supplement is a good cautionary choice, as the super-unsaturated oils always carry with them the risk of excessive free radical damage. It is always a sound practice, if you are getting accustomed to a supplement regime, to stop your vitamins every six weeks for a week to ten days; this will help to reveal persistent deficiency and to re-establish endogenous balance.

Foods naturally rich in omega 3 fat have the neutralizing anti-oxidants embedded within them. Salmon, for example, is orange because it's rich in the anti-oxidant beta carotene. This helps to minimize the depletion of endogenous anti-oxidants, and will help minimize oxidation of the highly unsaturated omega 3 fats. Antioxidants that we find naturally in foods are often not present in the fish oil supplements, but the antioxidants are sold separately.

There are some very good websites containing information designed to help people reverse the effects of excessive omega 6 in their diets and increase dietary intake of omega 3 fatty acids. These sites will help you to monitor your progress, and to calculate just where you are with your omega 6/ omega 3 nutritional balance. I highly recommend them if you are currently supplementing with fish oils and still eating refined vegetable oils high in omega 6 fatty acids. They are listed in the bibliography at the back of the book.

Most North Americans would benefit greatly from rebalancing their omega 3/ omega 6 ratios. In general, your long-term health will improve if you eat more fish, flaxseed oil and flax seeds, and eat a lot less mixed vegetable, safflower, sunflower, corn and soybean oils. And it is most important to recognise that the sheer quantity of food that North Americans typically consume at any one meal will amplify the negative affects of omega 6 fatty acids. So eat less!

---

7.   Sheila Innis, Ph. D., Director, Nutrition and Metabolism Research Program Child and Family Research Institute, UBC Canada.

8.   J. R. Hibbeln et al. 2007. Maternal seafood consumption in pregnancy and neurodevelopmental outcomes in childhood (ALSPAC study): an observational cohort study. *Lancet* 369 (9561)

CHAPTER 13
TRANS FATTY ACIDS

"Trans fat is even more harmful than saturated fat. When partially hydrogenated vegetable oil was first used in foods many decades ago, it was considered safe. Now that the studies have demonstrated partially hydrogenated oil is a major cause of heart disease, it should be phased our of food supply as rapidly as possible and replaced with more healthful oils."[9] (Golly, my Grandma knew all that!)

In Canada, it was stated that greater than 60% of the trans fat consumed comes from processed foods, and only 11% come from margarines. ... In contrast to Canada and the United States, the use of partially hydrogenated oils with trans fats is not widespread in European countries. *Dairy and animal fats are very often used in European countries, animal fats contribute - 40%-70% of total fat intake.* [10] (my italics)

What are trans fats?

Trans fats are formed by infusing hydrogen atoms into unsaturated liquid oils such as corn, soybean, safflower, sunflower or canola with a metal catalyst at extremely high temperatures. This is *hydrogenation*. If we use the caterpillar analogy, it's like welding little shoes onto our caterpillar's feet with burning hot iron or nickel prongs, then twisting the caterpillar's legs up vertically until they're perpendicular to their original position. Trans configuration fats can't move, wiggle or take off their hydrogen shoes and prepare for digestion. They are stable.

Trans fatty acids were a brilliant invention from the point of view of large-scale food producers; hydrogenation allowed them to make use of cheap remnants of oil left over from extraction, and also represented a way of increasing the shelf life of oils that oxidise. The use of trans fatty acids in place of other oils and fats also increased the shelf life of products they contained – but they now have to be removed from our food supply because they decrease the shelf life of those who eat them! Hydrogenation can be 'complete' or 'partial'.

Complete and partial hydrogenation

Complete hydrogentation will make the unsaturated oil completely saturated, with hydrogen at each carbon atom (lots of little shoes). The fat created will then behave like a saturated fat — though it is still *labelled* as an unsaturated fat because it started out as a *liquid* oil. Complete hydrogenation creates a very stable, heat tolerant fat that can be fried, baked, and put on shelves for a very long time. Until recently, hydrogenated fats were promoted to the consumer as 'unsaturated oils'; they were labelled as hydrogenated, but this was at a time when the consumer did not know what this meant – either chemically, or for their health. Complete hydrogenation also creates unnatural fragments of fatty acids that the body's enzyme system cannot recognize. And the metal catalyst — iron, copper, or nickel — remains as a residue in the fat it has been used to create. The human body does not need, and cannot use, artificial, manufactured hydrogenated fats.

Coconut and palm kernel oil are the only completely hydrogenated fats that do not pose a major health risk; this is because less than 10% of their profile is unsaturated to begin with, this 10% is predominately in the form of shorter chain fats. If you were a purest you wouldn't eat *any* hydrogenated products, but these two represent the least bad choices. The palmoleic fatty acid (this is a 16 carbon fat from palm oil with one double bond that makes it the unsaturated oil in palm oil) also responds in a relatively benign way to hydrogenation because it is simply transformed into the naturally occurring version of palm oil, and the body recognises this modified fat. Still, the natural versions of these fats are always preferable.

Partial hydrogenation occurs when the hydrogenation process is stopped before it has been brought to completion. Partial hydrogenation is a *random process* that creates an infinite variety and combination of trans fatty acids. The hydrogen atoms attach on opposite sides of the double bond of the oil and create a stable 'trans formed' molecule. (It's as if each caterpillar has one leg twisted perpendicular to its body.) The trans fatty acid molecule can no longer twist and turn like the original fatty acid in the unsaturated fat. Partially hydrogenated trans fats act like saturated fats because the trans configuration makes them stable, even though in partial hydrogenation they are still unsaturated. Trans-formed fats are technically "unsaturated", and they were promoted as such for several decades. Recall that the vegetable oils are made up of long chain unsaturated fatty acids; hydrogenation makes these long chain acids behave like saturated fatty acids by making them more stable.

The body contains no enzymes capable of disentangling these artificial trans fatty acids once they are ingested. In metabolism the trans fats of partial hydrogenation block out the functions of the other fatty acids in the natural cis configuration. They fit where unsaturated fatty acids would fit into cell membranes, but they don't do the work of unsaturated fatty acids. They can't attach oxygen, they can't respond to insulin, so that sugar is left to circulate in the blood, and they are inert – not communicating with other cells and systems. Artificial trans fatty acids have no place in the body's biochemistry, and to the extent that they are recognised by the body on the basis of their partial resemblance to functional fatty acids, they only cause harm.

Trans fatty acids compete for the same enzymes that are used to metabolise essential fatty acids. Trans fats compete with omega 3 and 6 fats for use by cell membrane receptors. Trans fats cause damage to cell membranes by short-circuiting their electric potential (this is what helps muscle cells contract). Trans fatty acids interfere with the production of prostaglandin, which governs ongoing cellular activity on a moment-by-moment basis. Molecules, atoms and their electrons have a specific structure and spatial arrangement in relation to one another. This creates the flow of energy that is the source of all life forces. When artificial molecules with the wrong shape, size, and properties – like trans fats – are introduced into the building blocks of the body, they simply don't fit as they should. The flow of energy and the transfer of energy are all but thrown off course. Life-sustaining functions, including heartbeat, mental acuity, co-ordination and cellular mitosis, are derailed and interrupted. The natural flow of energy becomes something more like static on a phone line. Life on a cellular level gets mixed up messages, and health and vitality are impaired. This process is incremental, over the course of a lifetime, slowly short-circuiting our genetic potential for good health. In short; trans fatty acids have been identified as a factor in many of the endemic health problems of modern North American society because of their detrimental affects at the cellular level.

The Jersey cow has 3 stomachs, or rumen, and can 'bio-hydrogenate' to form trans vaccenic fatty acids from unsaturated fatty acid that pass through them. These naturally occurring trans fatty acids are recognized by the body and do metabolise well, because they are produced in predictable amounts and configurations that the body can recognize. This cannot be said of the artificial trans fats found in margarine, shortening, hydrogenated vegetable oils, partially hydrogenated oils and all products made from these fats; typically, crackers, cookies, cereals, breads, condiments, boxed treats, and pastries have all been high in trans fatty acids. The government regulations controlling trans-fatty acids came only after the public outcry, and a boycott of products containing these harmful fats. Food manufacturers, especially in Canada, are to be commended for embracing the challenge and voluntarily labelling their products with a fatty acid profile even before it was mandatory in 2006. This helped Canadians become more aware of the trans-formed fats in food. It is amazing that otherwise-brilliant cardiologists insisted for so long on a trans fat rich diet for their patients' heart health; I have gone toe-to-toe with a couple of cardiologists to argue for butter and whole milk for a heart diseased client. And now, so many years later, my position has been proven to be correct. How many people were pushed further into the depths of disease by faulty diet recommendations?

The only genuinely 'bad' fats are those fats that have been chemically hydrogenated, partially hydrogenated, artificially polyunsaturated by the random insertion of double bonds, refined, processed with excessive heat, or solvent-extracted. The bad fat label should only be applied to those fats that interfere with the regular functioning of the body's biochemistry. And this occurs only when fats undergo chemical manipulation, so this category does not include any of the saturated fats; any fat eaten in its natural state, in the proper proportions, will have a health enhancing effect. The saturated fats of meat and dairy are essential for the human body. It is the refined, altered, rancid and processed oils, mixed vegetable oils, trans fats, and partially hydrogenated oils that have been directly linked to obesity, arthritis, arteriosclerosis, cellulite, high cholesterol and other degenerative health conditions, not saturated fat. So butter up, Buttercup!

A brief history of margarine

At the turn of the last century margarine consumption was less than 2 lbs per person per year. In 1990 margarine consumption peaked at 8.3 lbs per person per year. Is this the weapon of mass destruction? In North America, the media, governments and the private sector have spent the past 20 years bashing butter and extolling the virtues of margarine — and we've bought it! Literally! Oh we loooooooooove our margarine, because "it tastes like butter but it's not!".

Margarine was originally developed as a cheap non-perishable butter substitute for wartime troops, and for those who couldn't afford butter. But margarine achieved its largest market share in the 1990s, for quite different reasons, as the media portrayed saturated fats as bad for arteries and for overall health. Unsaturated fats, such as those found in modern margarines, were actually presented as *beneficial* for heart health – by manufacturers and the commercial media, by the Heart and Stroke Foundation, and by various governmental bodies. Physicians also lauded the merits of margarine, and butter was forbidden to heart patients and those with any perceived risk of heart disease.

Margarine's humble beginnings date back to 1869, when a French chemist named Hippolyte Mège-Mouriés was granted a patent for a butter substitute called 'oleomargarine'. The word margarine was derived from the Greek *margarites*, meaning 'pearl', because of the new substance's pearl-like sheen and colour. European commercial production of margarine was initiated in the 1870s by the Dutch company Jurgens. Mouries' margarine was made from beef tallow oleine, 10% milk, water, and udder tissue! The udder was of course added for extra flavour. This original recipe was not remotely as unhealthy as today's margarine products. At the time these *unhydrogenated* margarines were strictly regulated to ensure that they were indeed legally different from butter, but also to guarantee that they contained sufficient fat. Unlike margarine produced today, which typically has fat levels around 55%, margarine back then had to be 80% fat.

Then, in 1910, the commercial hydrogenation of vegetable oils began in the United States, originally as a way of making vegetable-oil candles (yum!). When this project was unsuccessful, the substance was reconstituted and repackaged as a substitute for lard, and Crisco hasn't looked back since – though from 1916-1920 soap-makers Procter and Gamble battled them over the hydrogenation patent. It wasn't until the 1930s that bleaching, neutralizing, deodorization, hardening, and fractioning began to be used to manipulate margarine's consistency and flavour. With all the new food technologies of the 1930s the original tallow based margarine was subject to de-vitamination (the removal of vitamins) in the course of ever more complicated manufacturing processes. Laws were then passed that required vitamins to be added *back* into margarines. The United Kingdom declared the modern margarine of the 1930s unfit for children because of its devitalized state.

Margarine continued to evolve through the decades, morphing from a simple and inexpensive butter substitute with an extended shelf-life in the 1870s, to a health food devoutly believed to protect our hearts a century later, to the present day margarine mayhem! Modern margarines are made largely from unsaturated oils (in their natural states or hydrogenated), water, lecithin and whey. After the trans fatty acid debacle, margarines are now trans fat free, and hydrogenation has been replaced by processes such as *interesterification,* by which fatty acids are redistributed on the glycerol to yield a product with different characteristics than the original. Interesterification usually involves oils being catalysed with sodium methoxide. Does that sound good for us?

Margarines are far less expensive than butter, and margarine can be left on the counter, or forgotten in the trunk of the car until next grocery day and still be edible. Butter, on the other hand, needs to be refrigerated or it will go rancid. The shelf-life of margarine is practically limitless; in terms of longevity, margarine wins hands down over butter.

Margarine in our home

I always tell the story of going home to bake cookies at Christmas time. My mother has 6 children and 3 stepchildren, so packing the pantry was serious business. She never let supplies get low. While searching the cellar pantry for more 'hard fat' I found a hard, bright yellow brick of margarine wrapped in wax paper. I couldn't believe my eyes; that pound of margarine must have been pushed to the back of the pantry and never rotated to the front of the line. How long has it been since margarine came wrapped in nothing but waxed paper? It was way back in the 1960s and 70s that paper wrappers were phased out and replaced by plastic tubs. This margarine was not in a bucket or plastic pail, just nice crisp wrappers of dusty, folded waxed paper. I remembered that yellow brick of ChefMaster margarine – it had always been there. "Mom," I yelled, "You have margarine down here that is 20 years old."

"Oh I do not!" she replied, and as she bounded down the stairs toward the pantry she yelled. "It's a new package." Then we launched into one of our nutrition issue face-offs. "Mom," I said, "That is no computer generated logo or font, and the dust on top of the package is just not new!" Mom hesitated, then grabbed the package out of my hand and said, "Oh it's still good!"

So we made the date squares. Was the margarine still good? Yes, Mom was right, because technically the margarine was still good. The margarine was stable, it hadn't gone rancid, it hadn't even melted – or if it had, it had hardened right back up again. The margarine was good enough, and my brothers happily gobbled up those tasty date squares. But my daughter Lucy and I only ate the pure butter shortbread cookies.

Modern margarines

When the news regarding trans fats hit the media there was a frenzied effort to shore up margarine's market share, and the new 'non-hydrogenated' spreads have flooded the supermarket shelves. These newer, trans fat-free margarines have higher water to fat ratios. The water used in the emulsion of margarine destroys the double bonds that may have survived the oils' processing. The double bonds are of course the 'health benefit' that unsaturated oils offer. When these double bonds are destroyed their metabolic breakdown is impeded. They are technically *not* trans fats, however their chemical configuration doesn't permit them to behave any better than a trans configuration fatty acid. Margarines are still made with blended, poor quality oils rich in omega 6 and insufficient in omega 3, and without any of the benefits of saturated butterfat. Any way you spread it, old oil made new again is still a rancid food product. Why would anyone eat this stuff?!

You can find countless charts that compare the levels of trans fatty acids in different types of margarines. The hard, solid bars of margarine have higher concentrations of trans fatty acids than the soft tub margarines. But in my view it is not remotely important to compare these worst of all evils. If you are concerned with your health, and especially if you want to make the best choices for your children, margarine of any type shouldn't even be considered. Ignore the graphs and charts! The advertising for modern margarines is astounding. Most of it wants to convince the consumer that the product is rich in omegas 3 and 6. But read the ingredient list closely; omega 6 will be the most abundant fatty acid, and *no one* in North America needs to supplement their diet with *more* omega 6. Do the right thing and just don't eat it.

Trans fatty acids and affects on health

Trans fatty acids and their equivalents can substantially increase blood triglyceride levels. Consistently elevated blood triglycerides levels represent a stage in the development of atherosclerotic plaque, mostly because of the inflammatory response that these trans fatty acids mediate. And there is a great deal of research concerning the relationship between trans fatty acids and cancer; though the increase in consumption of hydrogenated vegetable oil that parallels the increase in the incidence of cancer doesn't 'prove' causation, it could perhaps demonstrate a co-relation.

All in all, trans fatty acids are destructive substances that play havoc with the natural energy production that constitutes our life force. If there is a direct or indirect relationship between trans fatty acids and disease, and *absolutely no benefit* to their inclusion in our diet, then they simply have no place in our food supply... for anyone, even those who can't afford butter. There has to be another solution that benefits everyone.

9. Mary G. Enig. 2000. *Know Your Fats: The Complete Primer for Understanding the Nutrition of Fats, Oils, and Cholesterol.* Bethesda Press, pg. 11.
10. Nimal W. M. Ratnayake & C. Zehaluk. 2005. Trans Fatty Acids in Foods and Their Labelling Regulations, in Oi-Ming Lai and Casimir C. Akoh eds. *Healthful Lipids* AOCS Publishing, pg. 11.

Chapter 14

Cholesterol

A visit

I was immensely flattered when The Heart and Stroke Foundation telephoned to offer me a position as media spokesperson. Apparently they had heard about my passionate lectures on nutrition, and two of their representatives wanted to meet me. I had never avoided controversy in my career as a nutritionist; I felt the science of biochemical pathways to be my calling as much as my 'job'. And I was thrilled, but also a bit nervous, to finally be considered for such a high-profile public role.

The women arrived at my office mid-day and I offered water or tea as refreshment. There are always plenty of fresh organic nuts, fruits, seeds, carrots, peppers and eggs within arms reach of my desk; food is a wonderful ice breaker. The women commented on my slight figure – and whenever someone makes this observation I take the opportunity to inform them that my husband is an Italian chef. I think my response is largely defensive, since many women seem to simply assume that I have the appetite of a bird, or 'diet' obsessively, or have been blessed with a freaky rapid metabolism. On the contrary; my appetite is balanced to my energy expenditure, and my metabolism is driven by healthful food.

I launched into my standard inquiry; what foods did they eat? What time? How much sleep did they get? I was interviewing them about the status of their health. They seemed intrigued. Then out came the flip-chart and coloured markers and I buzzed around drawing lines and arrows, cells and cell membranes, all to illustrate my arguments that saturated fats are essential, and that a healthy metabolism is driven by plenty of food. The two women were overflowing with questions and requesting all sorts of nutrition advice. Then I dropped the bomb; the very margarine endorsed by the Heart and Stroke Foundation is made with saturated fat.

The two women fell silent. How could this product be made with a saturated fat, when decreasing dietary saturated fat was the mandate of the Heart and Stroke Foundation? In 'their' margarine, as in many others, the saturated fat palm oil is blended with unsaturated oils to make a spreadable semi-hard product. It's promoted as healthier than butter simply because it has less saturated fat than butter. And it does. But it has no beneficial short chain fats like butter, and no natural vitamins in it – just synthetic additives. It has poor-quality, highly processed vegetable oils blended with the palm oil, lots of water and no antioxidants, but plenty of artificial colour. Palm oil is about the only good thing in it! Perhaps it should be promoted as a margarine made with palm oil, the saturated fat that the body needs and benefits from, plus a lot of other junk.

The ladies were overwhelmed and we all took a breather to contemplate the invitation for Melissa to join the Heart and Stroke Foundation. Needless to say, my message that we should re-introduce wholesome saturated fats back into our diet is far too radical for the Heart and Stroke Foundation. Their fundamentalist creed calls for a diet high in unsaturated vegetable oils omega 6 and 9. Maybe another good position will come along.

The Heart and Stroke foundation didn't come by their motto "diet as the first line of defence against heart disease" all on their own; it represents their take on the diet-heart-lipid hypothesis that underlies so much mainstream nutrition policy. And so it is based on a body of conclusions stemming from cross-cultural research undertaken in the 1950s that seemed to link diets rich in saturated fat with a higher rate of heart disease. The Heart and Stroke Foundation therefore promotes diets that are low in total fat, low in saturated fat, and even lower in dietary cholesterol.

"The diet-heart hypothesis has been repeatedly shown to be wrong, and yet, for complicated reasons of pride, profit, and prejudice, the hypothesis continues to be exploited by scientists, fund-raising enterprises, food companies, and even government agencies. The public is being deceived by the greatest health scam of the century."[11]

Like George Mann, who wrote these words, I believe that it is only a matter of time before the merits of saturated fat and dietary cholesterol become accepted by the mainstream. The day will come when government publications will encourage us to cook with coconut, and to eat treats made with palm oil or butter, and to save the lard from our cooking. Since the population continues to struggle with weight and health issues, we will eventually be forced to face the truth; whole food, in its natural state, full of all varieties of fat, is the best way to achieve health and a sensible body weight. One day the Heart and Stroke Foundation will see things this way, too.

Cholesterol the good

Every person being encouraged or pressured to lower their cholesterol levels should know that cholesterol is present in every type of cell in their body. Cholesterol is a critical nutrient, without which the human body simply would not survive. Cholesterol is an unsaturated fat. It is one of the building blocks of nerve and brain tissues, and of the sex hormones oestrogen and testosterone. It builds the corticosteroid aldosterone, a hormone secreted by the adrenal glands to regulate fluid excretion, and cortisol, the hormone we secrete when under stress. Cholesterol is a precursor to vitamin D, the fat-soluble vitamin activated when ultraviolet light hits the skin. It is 7-dehydrocholesterol, a derivative of cholesterol, that reacts with ultraviolet light to form vitamin D3. D3 can also be provided by our diets; it is found mainly in meat and fish liver oil. (I think Grandma was right again with that tablespoon of cod liver oil.) The D3 is converted in the liver and kidneys to 25-hydroxycholecalciferol, and to 1,25-dihydroxylcholecaliciferol, which is the major circulating active form of Vitamin D. .

In the winter we produce less vitamin D3. And that's when it is important to seek out the dietary sources such as meat and fish oil. Egg yolks, butter and liver all have some vitamin D as well, as do fatty fish like salmon and mackerel. Non-homogenized full fat dairy milk also contains vitamin D. So the foods rich in vitamin D are on our prohibited list of foods. Vitamin D in its cholesterol base is essential in building and maintaining strong bones and teeth. It maintains a stable nervous system, normal heart action and proper blood clotting, all of which are related to proper calcium balance. Vitamin D is closely tied to the parathyroid glands that help regulate the hormones estrogen and cortisone. Because of its central role in bone formation, it is essential in consistent doses for children and the elderly. Though vitamin D is produced directly in the skin, it is released into the blood to reach other tissues.

It's a sad but true fact that every winter too many Canadians continue to slog away at their government approved low-fat diets, restricting animal fat and filling up on skim milk dairy products, all of which in their natural full-fat state *were* rich in vitamin D but, alas, no longer are. And these same health-conscious Canadians are meanwhile dutifully taking synthetic vitamin D supplements to boost their immunity and to make up for their lack of sun exposure, and their resulting low levels of endogenous vitamin D. If we just ate foods rich in real vitamin D there would be no need for synthetic replacements. This is another example of the many ways that, by avoiding whole foods on account of their cholesterol and fat content, we end up compromising our access to other essential symbiotic nutrients.

Cholesterol regulates serotonin receptors in the brain; these are the feel-good neurotransmitters which elevate our mood when activated. If an individual's cholesterol levels are regulated down to a point below what is normal for them, their mood is often sombre, progressing to depressive, and statistically significant increases in suicide and violent behaviour have been reported. My clients often voice their concern about depressed elderly parents that have been put on cholesterol medications. Research carried out at the University of Pittsburgh has shown a statistically significant increase in rates of death from violence and suicide among younger people with low cholesterol levels. And Professor Matthew Muldoon has established that low blood cholesterol levels are more common in criminals and in people with violent or aggressive conduct disorders. My Grandma knew that if my brothers were being particularly disorderly and aggressive, a good heavy meal of roast beef and whipped potatoes with cream and butter was enough to stop the fighting and obscenities, at least for a little while. She never yelled at them or us, she just quietly intervened with the call for meal time. And we would all sit at that round table with its drop-down table leafs and an embroidered tablecloth invariably covered in thick, stiff protective plastic. Maybe it was because she was hard of hearing that she never reacted to our infight-

The Benefits of Cholesterol

The body makes 1000mg grams of cholesterol every day!

Most reseach that compares the effect of two different dietary oils attributes the differences to the fatty acid composition. However, other components that are lower in concentration might have larger affects such as antioxodant concentration. Gurr pg 213

One pound of butter contains 1 gram of cholesterol
Udo pg 242

Infant metrx of cholesterol is fully developed before birth. Unlike long and short chain metrx which requires enzymes and further digestion. Infant LDL is higer to deliver protective cholesterol to developing tissues

Antioxidants

Heal arterial damage

Serotonin receptor in the brain

Cell membrane integrity

Lactobacillius, acidophillus increase metrx of cholesterol

Gurr pg 199

CHOLESTEROL

Corticosteroids
- Aldosteron (cortex)
- Cortisol (medulla)

Estrogen

Precursor to Vo to enhance Calcium assimilation

Testosterone

Integrity of gut mucosa -- faulty lining can lead to undigested foods (protien) getting into blood

Bile

Hypothyroidism couples high cholesterol - cholesterol floods the blood as an adaptive and protective mechanism to heal tissue damage and provide protective steroids

Lard 3500mg/g
Palm Oil 117mg/g

The less cholesterol you eat the more the body makes

Most experiments done on the detrimental effects of cholesterol have used oxidized, rancid cholesterol rather than pure cholesterol itself.
Luc Bucei
H. Gurr

ing, or expressed shock or disappointment. Or maybe she just knew that most family squabbles could be cured with a sated belly and a good nap. Nutrition feeds the brain, and the brain needs and thrives on cholesterol.

Many disease states can result from lowered cholesterol levels, or *hypocholesterolemia*. Cholesterol is the building block of our sex hormones, so lowered levels can have a negative impact on fertility and libido. Put together a lowered libido and an aggressive or depressive mood, and you have the makings of a serious negative feedback cycle; the less physical contact and intimacy a person receives, the more discontent and depressed they can become, potentially leading to aggressive outbursts – and who would want to have sex with someone like that, even if their libido *were* up to scratch? Cholesterol is required by every cell in the body, and people with unnaturally low levels often complain of muscular pain, as their tissue adjusts to these drastic changes. Medications that lower blood cholesterol levels to combat heart disease also lower cholesterol levels throughout the body. And this brings us to the crucial subject of cell membranes, and their dependence on adequate quantities of cholesterol.

Cholesterol builds and regulates cell wall membranes, helping to maintain the integrity of *all* cell walls. As Michael Gurr puts it: "The fluidity and stretch of cells is determined by the physical properties of lipids. Only cholesterol will allow animal membranes to function as required."[12] This quote summarises the complex and critical role cholesterol plays within all cells. Although it is not present in the mitochondrial membranes (the small compartments within cells that are responsible for cellular respiration), cholesterol can represent almost half the lipid component of other cell membranes. Cholesterol's integration into the lipid bi-layer allows it to influence cell membrane properties in complex fashion. Low-molecular-weight solutes can sometimes wreck havoc on the internal milieu of a cell, leading to potential malfunction; cholesterol binds with phospholipids to help keep these solutes out of the cell. Cholesterol actually disrupts the interactions between the longer chain fatty acid tails, which enhances membrane fluidity. This is an important function, and nutrition professionals always use this unsaturated fat fluidity as a positive for cell membranes. But it is actually the cholesterol that keeps long chain fatty acids from getting tangled, and disrupting cellular flow. Cholesterol virtually acts as a microcompartmental wall within cells, providing a way to spatially organize the pathways of cellular metabolism. Essentially, cholesterol has the ability to increase cellular membrane fluidity while decreasing unwanted permeability. This is a good thing for cellular health, and cellular health and stability are the foundations of optimum general health. We are made of cells.

Cholesterol is a vital and abundant *antioxidant*. As discussed in chapter ten, antioxidants neutralize the free radicals that contribute to disease by damaging cells. Antioxidants are part of the enzyme system that helps protect against environmental and metabolic toxins. Things like pesticides, plastics, smog, unsaturated fats and cigarette smoke can cause potent free radical damage. Just as hydrogen peroxide destroys bacteria and parasites, anti-oxidants protect our cells, and cholesterol is one of those crucial cell guardians. It helps to neutralize ongoing environmental damage at a cellular level.

---

11. George V. Mann. 1993. Coronary Heart Disease: the Dietary Sense and Nonsense pg. 1 (Dr. Mann was a participating researcher in the original Framingham Massachusetts study.)
12. Michael L. Gurr. 1999. Lipids in Nutrition and Health: A Reappraisal. pg. 15

CHAPTER 15
A BRIEF HISTORY OF CHOLESTEROL

Discovery

Cholesterol and its role in the body are not new objects of enquiry. Biologists have been searching for the biochemical mechanism that explains the formation of fatty streaks and atherosclerotic plaque – the first form in which cholesterol was observed – since at least as long ago as 1852, when Karl Rokitansky, professor of Pathology at the University of Vienna, first described arterial lesions. Rokitansky had been conducting over 2000 autopsies a year, and this experience ensured that he understood the full range of variations, healthy and unhealthy, that human organs could present. He proposed an 'injury hypothesis' to explain the arterial plaque that would build up not just in the heart, but throughout the body; he believed that cholesterol adhesions developed due to injury at the site. The German scientist Rudolf Virchow first noted atherosclerosis in 1856. He believed that very low-grade injury to the artery wall resulted in a type of inflammatory insudate (fluid swelling within the wall), which caused plasma constituents to build up.

The opposing theory, that cholesterol *caused* arterial plaque build-up, was later proposed by Nikolai N. Anitschkow, a pathologist working at the Military Medical Academy in St. Petersburg. He demonstrated that feeding rabbits sunflower oil and cholesterol induced vascular lesions that closely resembled human atherosclerosis. His work was criticized on the basis that rabbits, being exclusively herbivorous, likely had no mechanism to deal with excessive concentrations of blood cholesterols. Today we might also wonder whether rabbits have the anti-oxidant resources to deal with all that sunflower oil.

Nevertheless, the connection he suggested had supporters in the decades that followed. His original research was repeated by organic chemist David Kritchevsky, who published his results in the American Journal of Physiology in July 1954. Kritchevsky's study, "Effect of Cholesterol Vehicle in Experimental Atherosclerosis," studied the relationship in animal subjects between high-cholesterol diets and subsequent development of atherosclerosis. It concluded that dietary cholesterol levels affect the development of heart disease. This study is still often cited. In 1951 John W. Gofman, an MD and PhD in physics at the University of California, San Francisco, published the first low-fat, heart-healthy cook book. (Though it should also be noted that in 1825 the French chef Jean Anthelne Brillat-Savain had published *The Physiology of Taste,* which among other things outlined why fat is essential for human health. Who knew that this topic was already a matter of controversy so long ago!)

Cholesterol: the enemy within?

William Stamler and Ancel Keys were the driving forces behind population studies in the 1950s and 1960s that set out to connect dietary animal fat and cholesterol with incidence of heart disease. Meanwhile, the first paper of the famous Framingham Heart Disease Study was published in the American Journal of Public Health in 1957. The study supported the contentions that heart disease was more prevalent in males, that blood pressure increased risk, and that dietary cholesterol specifically increased the risk of coronary heart disease. Weight also was implicated in these first results, but smoking was not. Keys explained that dietary saturated fats 'stick' to arteries and that unsaturated fats are fluid and help to decrease the rigidity, and hence potential occlusion, of artery cell walls. His theory that dietary fat raises blood cholesterol levels, and so gives rise to heart disease, unambiguously supported the emerging paradigm that saturated fats and cholesterol should be avoided to ensure optimum health and freedom from heart disease. This was the 'diet-heart lipid hypothesis'.

Dissenters from Keys' work argued that its conclusions involved a circumvention of scientific method. And the evidence supporting his theories remained stubbornly ambiguous; the scientific community couldn't reach any consensus on the relationship between dietary cholesterol and heart disease. In the end, the issue was never settled in the court of science, on the basis of scientific enquiry and an accumulation of research that supplanted or confirmed existing theories. Instead, it was settled in a US Senate Committee! That's right, the official guidelines for your nutritional health weren't established by clever and enthusiastic scientists, with new research debunking old theories and extending the breadth of human knowledge; they were decided by politicians. The original research might have been carried out by brilliant scientific minds, but in the absence of conclusive research to implicate dietary cholesterol it was the Senate 'Select Committee on Nutrition and Human Needs', led by George McGovern – a smart politician but no scientist – that decided which research would shape the American people's diet and curb the steady increase in diseases seen as nutrition-related.

In the years leading up to 1977, several hundred million dollars were spent trying to definitively correlate the consumption of fat to rates of heart disease. Five major studies, (the Seven Countries studies, LCR, the Nurses Health Study, the Framingham Massachusetts Heart Study and 'Mr. Fit') despite the $110 million dollars they collectively cost, didn't actually reveal any such link. A sixth study, examining the use of drug therapy intervention, did show that lowering cholesterol deceased heart disease. Fair enough, but this study was not the equivalent of the dietary cholesterol studies, and did not address the relationship between diet and disease that they never managed to clarify; why were these clumps of cholesterol there in people's arteries in the first place? It was the administrators of the National Institute of Health who made the leap of faith, concluding that if cholesterol-lowering drug therapy ameliorated heart disease then this pretty much meant that dietary cholesterol must make it worse, even in the absence of scientific data to prove this relationship. It was thought that dietary cholesterol research would eventually establish the expected link between fat and heart disease.

So it was that in January 1977 the US Senate report *Dietary Goals for the United States* set forth objectives aimed at reducing the intake of fat, the "greasy killer". Despite continued disagreement within the scientific community about what constitutes healthy eating, and about which eating patterns contribute directly to disease, and despite the arguments of outright dissenters to the low-fat 'consensus', the floodgates had opened, and official nutrition advice poured out in ever-increasing volumes, now with a stamp of approval from the United States Senate. This advice established and reinforced the paradigm that remains firmly entrenched to this day; dietary saturated fat and cholesterol cause heart disease. Cholesterol research has engaged the minds and the laboratories of eminent biologists for a very long time, but there is a long way to go before we completely understand cholesterol's mechanisms. Its role in the body is not as simple as the current theories explaining it to the public make out. There is more to be learned, and medicating it out of our blood stream is not the definitive solution.

The history of heart disease diagnosis and its link to cholesterol

The ability to accurately diagnose heart disease has made fumbling progress since the turn of the last century; the condition has a long history of being misdiagnosed, under-diagnosed and group diagnosed, all of which have skewed historical statistics on the prevalence of heart disease in our society.

First established in 1893 by the International Statistical Institute at a meeting in Chicago, the International Classification of Disease (ICD) was a register for codifying diseases and tracking their patterns and prevalence, in order to improve diagnosis and to supply data for medical research. Its records show that there has always been a recognition that heart disease is not a single disorder, but the result of a complex and varied etiology. We now know that some causes of heart disease are congenital, that some relate to damage suffered by the heart muscle, and that others are a result of inflammation and suppressed immunity. Heart disease can also be related to viral and bacterial disease. The classification of heart disease at one time included *angina pectoris, pericarditis, acute endocarditis*, and organic diseases of the heart. Of all of these, only angina pectoris is related to heart disease. This suggests that doctors knew little about heart disease, or disagreed concerning its classification and the symptomatology to be included in this classification. This ongoing disagreement would inevitably skew the patterns of diagnosis for heart disease.

Our understanding of the complexities of heart disease has continued to evolve to this day, and the search for a consensus concerning what it is, and what it is not, continues. As the ICD went forward (it is now in its tenth revision) there were changes to the classification of heart disease. There was the inclusion of coronary artery disease under the angina pectoris classification, which led to the establishment of a 'disease' called coronary heart disease. This led to a substantial increase in the diagnosis rate of heart disease in the 1940s, largely due to this classification change rather than to any actual increase in the incidence of disease.

By the 1950s, when the use of the electrocardiograph was increasing exponentially, the reporting of coronary heart disease as a cause of deaths increased again. The ICD's ongoing revision of what constituted heart disease continued to alter the apparent prevalence of coronary heart disease. One of the major revisions was in 1962, when hypertension was lumped into the coronary heart disease category.

This change, in the 8th revision of the ICD, had a fundamental impact on Framingham heart study statistics. The Framingham Heart Study was the first large population-based study to track the impact of dietary cholesterol on heart disease. Its 1960 results appear to support the hypothesis that decreased cholesterol intake correlates with decreased incidence of heart disease. However there is reason to believe that the classification amendment could have influenced the statistical outcome. The addition of hypertension produced another dramatic increase in the reported incidence of coronary heart disease, giving the appearance of a sudden heart disease epidemic. For ICD revision 9, published in 1978, it was decided to remove hypertension from the Coronary Heart Disease category, which then presented a statistical decrease. What a roller coaster ride! We know that the heart can develop disease; we know that many people die of a diseased heart. What we do not know unequivocally is whether saturated fat and cholesterol are primary causal factors in the heart disease epidemic.

It's clear that there is a complex interplay between the official categorisation of diseases, the patterns of diagnosis identifying diseases and causes of death, and the scientific explanations linking diseases to causal factors. With respect to diagnosis; within the medical practice of western and westernised cultures there is a shared assumption that death for many people will be a result of the cumulative breakdown of more than one function within the body, while death certificates, and the statistics that are generated from their contents, generally only indicate *one* cause of death. Recognition of this fact, and its implications, led researchers Drs.

George D Lundberg and Gerhard Voigt to explore its possible significance. They demonstrated statistically that there are distinct preferences for particular 'presumptive diagnoses' – the reasons *presumed* to be the cause of death – among the physicians of a given country. Lundberg and Voight demonstrated that when completing death certificates, North American doctors ascribe death to coronary heart disease 50% more often than Norwegian doctors and 30% more often than British doctors. The patterns of official causes of death reported by physicians thus varied widely from one country to the next, but they also demonstrated a strong uniformity within a given country. The diets of these nations are similar, with few significant variations. So the country a person happens to die in will influence the presumed cause of death entered on their death certificate, with national preferences for one particular factor out of those that have contributed to death. This in turn will affect the mortality statistics compiled from the results of death certificates.

If North American doctors do over-diagnose heart disease as a cause of death, then perhaps there isn't an epidemic at all. If there really isn't a heart disease epidemic, but only a skewed pattern of diagnosis, then all the dietary changes we're being encouraged to adopt, and most of the restrictions being imposed on food manufacturers, are for naught. If Voight and Lundberg are correct concerning physicians' national or cultural partialities for particular diseases, then it is possible that our prevention protocol for heart disease is misdirected. If that were the case then the battle against fats, cholesterol, and heart disease would not be the first line of defence against mortality. If we are not dying of heart disease at rates like North American death certificates assert, then it stands to reason that the dietary recommendations with which we are combating *heart* disease might be pointlessly causing *other* disease states to flourish.

The 'rate of risk scale'

"37% of all Canadians over 40 years of age take some type of cholesterol lowering medication. Since 1990 incidence of cardiovascular disease is still unchanged. 80% of heart attack victims have normal cholesterol blood levels." [13]

40% of heart attacks occur in individuals without atherosclerosis. This is an important statistic, and one that all cholesterol lowering patients should be made aware of. This means there is no cholesterol-rich plaque clogging the arteries of these heart attack victims. Furthermore, heart disease as we define it claims more lives among the elderly than any other disease does. Atherosclerosis (heart disease) is a deterioration of arteries and as our population ages it follows that heart disease will inevitably increase. Atherosclerosis affects all populations throughout the world. Drs. Thomas Dawber and William Kannel, who knew these facts concerning heart disease, were not deterred.

1961 saw the publishing of Dawber and Kannel's landmark study "Factors of Risk in the development of Coronary Heart Disease". It was in this paper that the term 'risk factors' was coined – to quantify an individual's chances of developing heart disease. Their research seemed to show that cholesterol levels up to 182mg/dl (milligrams per decilitre) are associated with a .54/1000 risk of coronary heart disease. This means that of a thousand people with cholesterol levels in this range, less than one will have the related form of heart disease. Needless to say, this is not a very significant rate. For cholesterol levels between 182 and 244mg/dl the rate of risk increases from .054% to .184% (or one in 543 – still not a significant rate, though more than three times the rate of the lower-cholesterol group.

This study was influential in two subsequent developments. First, since high blood cholesterol was implicated in heart disease, the belief paradigm of 'lipid hypothesis' proponents led them, without justification, to assume that this higher cholesterol level simply *caused* heart disease – something that the figures did not prove. This led proponents of the lipid hypothesis to encourage people to aim for extremely low levels of circulating cholesterol. Second, it gave lipid hypothesis proponents the opportunity to emphasise the *relative* rate of heart disease, even though in the scientific community it was, and is, controversial to represent rates of death and disease in this way.

Even though doing so constituted what science writer Gary Taubs has called "soft science", the risk scale was condensed, with the percentage fractions converted into a "risk range scale" that ran from "one" to "three". When these cholesterol ranges are plotted on this scale, the associated risk of developing heart disease can be represented as a 240% increase, while the fact that this represents an increase from a 1 in 1852 chance to a 1 in 543 chance is obscured. This scale 'zooms in' on the difference, and hides the fact that both numbers, and both risks, are very small, especially when viewed in the context of the inevitable toll that age takes on the heart and arteries, and that this is a rate of disease, not heart attack or death. The rate of risk scale was very easy for doctors to explain to patients, and gave patients a way of interpreting the 'relative risk' of their developing heart disease.

In retrospect, it seems clear that the rate of risk scale discouraged patients from learning the normal range thresholds for cholesterol throughout the human life cycle. And it has been said that the risk scale sent cholesterol research off on a new trajectory, shutting down whole avenues of investigation. The rate of risk scale helped ramp up the increasing paranoia about blood cholesterol, because everyone would know someone who was 'at risk', and inevitably on 'preventative' medication. Everyone was paying attention to cholesterol.

But this scale had critics from its inception. Risk factor, as Gary Taubes and lipid biologist Michael Gurr often take the opportunity to point out, is not even remotely connected to *mortality*. No matter where we all fall on the rate of risk heart disease scale, and no matter how many new heart disease medications we take, and no matter how many dietary changes we embrace, one thing has not changed: the *rate of occurrence* of first heart attacks (as opposed to second or third heart attacks) is the same as it has always been. As a nation we are collectively having just as many first heart attacks; they are essentially not being prevented. Emergency care is more timely and effective, and more people are surviving the first and even second or third heart attack. But despite this, and despite all the new medications and all the dietary changes, first heart attacks are still occurring at the same rate as ever. But the rate of risk scale was a powerful and persuasive tool; there were no complex numbers or percentages to interpret, and so dogmatic dietary advice could be presented in terms essentially designed to scare patients for (what most doctors believed was) their own good.

Despite criticism of the rate of risk heart disease scale, in 1961 its popularity led the American Heart Association (AHA) to announce official recommendations for those with measurable coronary heart disease 'risks'. The AHA recommended that those deemed 'at risk' decrease saturated fats and dietary cholesterol, and replace both with substantial amounts of polyunsaturated fat. The cholesterol ranges charted by the risk scale encompassed a large percentage of the population, and the AHA's dietary recommendations started to address and affect a lot of people. As a follow-up to the AHA's 1961 recommendations, its 1964 recommendations, based on assumptions extrapolated from the Framingham Heart Study, advised that all Americans should adhere strictly to the 'Prudent Diet'. The Prudent Diet was an ascetic and controversial diet based on corn oil, cold cereal, chicken, and margarine. It was to be adopted alongside continued adherence to the earlier AHA recommendations to decrease total fat intake and substitute unsaturated for saturated fats. Cholesterol, saturated fat, red meat, eggs, butter, cheese, and spirits were all now 'forbidden fruit', as it were, for the American people.

Many pediatricians fervently opposed the Prudent Diet recommendations, as children's growth is dependant on fat and cholesterol. Mother's milk is 50% cholesterol!!! (Apparently it's quite sweet too, as my brother can attest. He accidentally took a gulp of my younger sister's refrigerated breast milk – not something brothers are encouraged to do. He'll kill me for writing this.) Mothers everywhere were encouraged to kick the butter 'habit' and to spread margarine instead. By now shortening wasn't just being promoted as the only fat capable of making a flaky pie crust; it also made pie more healthful.

Skim milk, later joined by low-fat cheese, low fat yoghurt, and on and on, was to become the norm for children and adults alike, despite the fact that children were not yet overweight – this was a problem that emerged in the 1980s and has continued into the new millennium. The subject of childhood dietary recommendations has continued to be mired in controversy. In 2008 the American Academy of Pediatricians released guidelines recommending low-fat milk for one-year-olds and cholesterol lowering medication for children as young as eight. These are drastic and unprecedented recommendations, which seem to reflect nothing but blind obedience to the crude, simple-minded belief that saturated fat and dietary cholesterol are solely responsible for the epidemic of degenerative heart disease and obesity.

The American Heart Association diet recommendations were further revised in 1968; the recommended cholesterol intake was reduced from 500mg to an frugal 300mg per day. The proportion of total daily calories eaten in the form of fats was to decrease from 37% to just 30-35%. In the 1968 revisions it was recommended that fat intake reflect an equal balance of saturated fats and monounsaturated/polyunsaturated fat. These recommendations for fat balance were included because of growing concern about the dominance of polyunsaturated fat in the North American diet. Polyunsaturated fats were known even then to increase cancer risk. This is largely because unsaturated fats oxidise and initiate free radical proliferation, as we discussed in chapter 7.

A decade later, in 1977, the US Senate Select Committee on Nutrition and Human Needs released *Dietary Goals for the United States*. The report stated six goals. The first was to *increase* carbohydrate consumption to 55-60% of caloric intake – though there was little distinction made concerning the quality of the carbohydrates that were to be consumed. North Americans had already increased their carbohydrate consumption to 60 pounds per person per year, and were eating an average of 30 pounds a year of high fructose corn syrup, as compared to *none at all* at the turn of the 20th century. These recommendations defined a diet that had Americans eating an extra 400 calories per day, despite their diets being lower in fat. And these calories have stayed with us since then, even increased somewhat. Endocrinology was not as advanced in 1977 as it is today, and the nature and functions of insulin, like those of dietary cholesterol, were not yet completely understood. Research on the effects of insulin, blood sugar, and weight gain on health couldn't be used as an argument against the recommended high-carbohydrate, low-fat diet.

But my Grandma knew the perils of a starch-rich breakfast. When everyone else was pouring skim milk over their cold cereal and eating it with orange juice and dry toast, Mindy and I got to fry our own baloney for breakfast. That heavy iron skillet sat securely on top of the gas flame and we moved the triangular slices all over the pan, just like Grams showed us. Then when everything was good and crisp we flipped it; it sure felt like we were cooking. It was a stove and a flame and a heavy iron pan. My mother hated to watch this, but Grams was pragmatic about it all. If a spark of grease spat out at us she would kiss it better. It worked, and we never cried making baloney hats. And of course we ate them with sliced tomatoes on the side; if the tomatoes were still green she fried those too!

The McGovern report called for an overall *reduction* in fat consumption to 30% of caloric intake, with saturated fats limited to 10%. Sugar was to be limited to 15% of calories, cholesterol intake to 300mg per day (half of what is normally needed by someone of balanced body weight who metabolises cholesterol normally) and salt to 3 grams per day. This clearly represented a call for Americans to eat more fruit, bread, vegetables, cereals, grains, poultry and fish, and to reduce their consumption of meat, eggs, butter, cheese and whole milk.

The report was also a very good marketing tool for all the new products that would soon be promoted to 'decrease the risk' of heart attack. It would be a few decades before the general public caught up and understood that the foods promoted to decrease risk of heart disease might be too dense in refined carbohydrates to do any good – might in fact even increase blood cholesterol profiles, because they drive up triglyceride levels as the body struggled to cope with overconsumption of carbohydrates. And never mind that so many products were promoted as 'cholesterol free' versions of familiar foods, when the original food had no cholesterol in the first place; this sort of doubletalk might be meaningless as a description of the foods in question, but it says a great deal about the relationship between science and economics underlying too much of the 'healthy food' industry.

The hysteria about cholesterol and heart disease was in full force. The average North American was by now only too aware that lifestyle choices, especially diet, and above all the amount and types of *fats* they ate, were going to have an impact on their health. This diet-centric, fat-phobic paradigm is still dominant today; instead of being proactive about their health by exercising more and eating less, North Americans have focused on simply modifying their diets as directed, by eliminating saturated fats and replacing them with unsaturated fats and trans fatty acids from hydrogenated fats. We are not eating less fat today, just different types of fat, many of them fake or made from inferior products. And we are eating more flour-based and sugary foods, which we now know have a deleterious affect on insulin regulation, which in turn affects blood triglyceride levels, ultimately leading to greater risk of diabetes and obesity.

The opportunity to encourage North Americans to become active, healthy eaters was wasted, as the Senate report's main message encouraged Americans to focus on a single category of nutrient, and to avoid it at any cost. This deflected attention from the real issues – being more active and eating less food – and encouraged a passive approach to improving 'lifestyles', as communicated by public service messages on the televisions that we sat watching while we ate more and more of the new 'healthy' foods. North Americans dutifully replaced treats containing saturated fats with the same treats made with other fats, or had it done for them by the manufacturers of commercial food products. There was never anything to be gained from this one-dimensional approach to heart disease, even if it *had* been based on good science.

Cholesterol consensus versus cholesterol dissent

The Cholesterol Consensus Conference in 1984 released a final report that declared 200mg/dl (milligrams per decilitre) of cholesterol to be the new lower limit defining 'at risk' individuals, despite the arguments of opponents who suggested that 240mg/dl should be the level that distinguished health from 'health problem'. Drs. Oliver, Grundy, Mann, Mensink, and Katan, collectively voiced their concern regarding the new recommendations; they disapproved of the policy of...

"...encouraging Americans to decrease cholesterol to 200mg/dl in view of the fact that many disorders derive from many kinds of deficiencies, as well as an over-production of normal body substances. It is incredible that the alliance encourages essentially unlimited reductions in blood cholesterol without seriously addressing scientifically the issue of deficiency."[14]

Imagine: there are scientists out there today who actually believe we can be cholesterol deficient! In fact, it's all too easy to become deficient in cholesterol, when cholesterol-lowering medications are thrown into the mix along with a low fat diet and the specific avoidance of cholesterol-rich foods. There is no definitive scientific evidence establishing that everyone is able to synthesize enough cholesterol, an essential component of health, to meet their needs. This alone is reason enough for low-level cholesterol recommendations not to be promoted, especially to a general population that has no elevated risk of heart disease.

But opponents of these drastically low cholesterol recommendations are still not being heard. Only in the last few years has a more open-minded approach emerged within the scientific community at large. Research funding for studies on the effects of fat and cholesterol has only just begun to flow. But it *has* begun. Schneider Children's Hospital on Long Island, the Philadelphia V.A. Hospital, and the Universities of Pennsylvania and Colorado are all investing in research about higher fat, higher cholesterol diets. The dissenters are there, and hopefully their message will soon be heard in the mainstream. The victims of the obesity and diabetes epidemics, and of the low-fat low dietary cholesterol regime that hasn't improved a single thing, are literally dying for the results of the research. I predict that we will one day ask ourselves how, as thinking adults who cared about what we ate, we ever believed that eating fake foods, altered fats and refined carbohydrates, or taking drugs that shut down our bodies' production of an essential substance like cholesterol, could be the road to improved health!

Cholesterol and the food industry

In 1938, the American Congress passed the Food Drug and Cosmetic (FDC) Act, a wide-ranging bill that included provisions allowing for government-mandated standardisation of food quality. This law was meant to prevent new food products from getting to market that were formulated to be *low* in cholesterol and fat! Decades later, the nation's growing angst over dietary cholesterol meant that the law, put into place to protect consumers against imitation foods, had to be re-evaluated. Ironically, the most health-conscious North Americans had come, over time, to be those most willing to accept fake foods in their pantry, even though the original law had been formulated so as to safeguard authentic foods from being confused with 'imitation' foods made from inferior products.

Peter Barton Hutt, a food lawyer in Washington D. C., became the US Food and Drug Administration's Chief Counsel in 1971. Hutt piloted the FDA through the legalities of establishing the new 'imitation policy' that became law in 1973. The new policy was designed to embrace 'advances in food technologies', and to free manufacturers from the dilemma of having either to comply with 'outdated standards' or to market their food products labelled unappealingly as 'imitation'. Once this law was passed, new products flooded the market. Nutritionally inferior food products could be sold right next to the authentic versions, which would inevitably be more expensive.

This policy fuelled the rapid expansion of an industry geared towards producing fake, adulterated, processed foods. Low-fat, non-fat, light, cholesterol free foods became our new healthy foods. Yoghurt, a food once the preserve of health food fanatics, was stripped of its valuable fats and packed full of starch, guar gum binders and sugar. This wasn't enough for some people, and yoghurt food products were introduced with 0% fat and artificial sweeteners in place of the sugar. A once balanced whole food, with near equal portions of fat, protein and carbohydrate was transformed into an unrecognisable imitation of itself.

Blinded by science, we no longer felt we had to be able to recognize what ingredients made up a food. Foods were literally created in laboratories. The grocery store was transformed into a carnival of consumption, and foods that were once considered treats were put on the breakfast table – often in their new guise as 'healthy' alternatives! (To what?!?) Increasingly, foods were marketed and purchased on the basis of a single nutrient that they contained, or didn't contain, and we stopped focusing on diet as a whole and began to buy foods according to a stream of shifting nutritional fads. But alongside this descent into obedient ill-health, there has always been an opposing body of research, which has recognised modified foods as nutritionally unsound, and as potentially contributing to disease. I hope one day our food policy is rebuilt on the basis of this recognition.

Snack foods

Snacking was once reserved for impatient, super-active young children when they returned from a busy day of school and play. But at some point snacks started to become meals in their own right, for all ages, as cooking and family meals gradually became relics of a bygone era. The food industry enthusiastically 'catered' to this demand, by creating all manner of foods that we hadn't even known existed. And of course all these foods were marketed as being good for our health, and the perfect answer to the nutritional demands of growing children. Snack foods became a substitute for eating a balanced meal. Snacks were formulated without cholesterol, or saturated and trans fats. They were instead made with 'heart healthy' unsaturated oils. Of course food colouring, sodium, high fructose corn syrup, and the residue from refined carbohydrates were standard ingredients in these commercial foods; but none of that seemed to matter as long as unsaturated oils were used. Children were being raised understanding that a snack was a food that came from a box, and not a simple piece of fruit or cheese. And now, snack foods constitute an industry so large that it seems to support half the television channels in North America, and to have become a central part of our collective existence. That raw hunger that active kids experience started to melt away as snack foods became ubiquitous; always available and always encouraged. Mealtimes have became microwave moments squeezed into the spaces where packed schedules intersect. For many of us they are no more than a ghostly shadow of what family meals had been for centuries.

The 2007 Morgan Stanley report on snacking showed an exponential increase in snacking since the 1980s, and it is still climbing today. There's no sort of food that lends itself to packaging and branding better than the 'snack' – the epitome of nutrition defeated by commercial interests. Is our children's health being compromised simply because we don't have the sense to see that the way we've changed our eating habits is far more convenient for the corporate food industry than it is for us and our busy lives?

13. "Reliability of a presumptive diagnosis in sudden unexpected deaths in adults. " JAMA, 1979, 242,2328-2330.)
14. Barry Goldman, Pharmacist. April 2008, Life Peak magazine
15. Russell L. Smith, with Edward R. Pinckney, 1993 – The Cholesterol Conspiracy. pg. 94

CHAPTER 16

SERUM CHOLESTEROL

Get your stories straight!

In his 2001 article "The Soft Science of Dietary Fat", Gary Taubes presents an overview of many years of cholesterol research, and points out that blood cholesterol levels in the range of 200 to 240 mg/dl were once deemed quite healthy and normal, with *no elevated risk of heart disease*. Of course science certainly has the prerogative, even the responsibility, to alter its paradigms and assumptions in the light of new research. But there is a clear lack of consensus about what constitute healthy blood cholesterol levels, and Taubes' overview of earlier research suggests that levels now deemed to be putting people 'at risk' were once considered normal, and that levels now considered healthy were once considered low. Remember; the idea that cholesterol levels could be too *low* has been off the map for a long time now. Has this ratcheting downwards of recommended healthy levels reflected emerging science, or simply a stubborn desire to defend the lipid hypothesis down to the last cardiac patient? (In a hole? Dig harder!)

Dr. William Lands' contribution to the 2005 book 'Healthful Lipids', goes into extensive detail concerning the essential role of all cholesterols in the blood, and argues that removing them with drug therapies is only removing a symptom and not its cause. Lands asks, "Does removal of clinical signs of heart disease (LDL) remove the underlying nutritional imbalances (O6 to O3 ratios) that cause people to develop disease?" [16]

Lands' perspective is that of a dissident. He argues that an excessive consumption of polyunsaturated omega 6 fats, along with refined carbohydrates, actually *causes* blood cholesterol to increase. So why do many 'first time' low saturated fat dieters sometimes present lower blood cholesterol levels? According to Land, the polyunsaturated oils that get substituted into a diet for the saturated fats will be used to build cell membranes, changing the stability of cells. Cholesterol is then drawn *out* of the blood and into all the tissues in order to restore the fluidity and stability of cells. Returning *tissue* cholesterol levels back to a normal (healthy!) level results in a decrease in *blood* cholesterol levels. Remember, from the earlier section on cholesterol and cell membranes, that the cholesterol in a membrane 'controls permeability while maintaining stability.' A cell will always try to achieve this homeostasis, and it does so by taking up cholesterol from the blood. Eventually the liver will likely start to produce more cholesterol to meet the demands of the hungry cells, rendering this type of highly unsaturated diet ineffective.

Eventually pretty well all of us will be confronted with the suggestion that we should medicate and diet away our rising cholesterol levels. It is important to understand a little bit about the roles played by the different cholesterols in the blood *before* it is our turn to deal with the issue. Here is an overview of the different blood cholesterols and how they function in the body. They work in tandem, and in most of the population they are perfectly synchronized.

Cholesterol is a fat – though unlike triglycerides and fatty acids, cholesterol is not an energy-producing nutrient. It is a 27 carbon acetate fragment made from excess sugars, alcohol, fat and dietary cholesterol. Because it is not used for energy it is eventually eliminated intact through the biliary system, a process that entails the use of bile stored in the gallbladder and moved through bile ducts. Some of the cholesterol is immediately excreted into the bile ducts, and some is converted into bile acids prior to entering the bile. Most bile acids are 55% neutral cholesterol.

The cholesterol-to-bile acid transformation involves adding other molecules to enhance the cholesterol/bile's water solubility. Bile itself is a fluid secreted by the liver and poured into the intestine, in order to produce an alkaline reaction in the intestine that aids in the emulsification and absorption of fats and helps prevent their incomplete digestion or putrefaction. Intestinal health is very important for efficient fat digestion. Bile is made of bile acids and pigments (that's why your poo is green if you aren't using the bile properly), cholesterol and mucin, which is the chief constituent of mucus. Bile and cholesterol are closely related. Bile salts returning to the liver from the intestine decrease the formation of an enzyme that converts cholesterol to bile acids, thus leading to increased cholesterol excretion.

HDL and LDL

High-density lipoprotein (HDL) is constructed with a little bit of cholesterol (about 19%) in its centre, surrounded by about 50% *apolipoprotein*. (Apolipoproteins are proteins whose role is to combine with lipids to form lipoprotein). Low-density lipoprotein (LDL) is the opposite – it's about 47% cholesterol, surrounded by just a thin 21% layer of proteins, and is destined for use by parts of the body that need more cholesterol. The proteins are important because they enable the lipid molecule to travel in the viscous blood. Recent research shows that these protein fractions are not inert vessels, but are responsible for how and where the cholesterol bundle will be received by receptors throughout the body. Different cells of the body have affinity for different apolipoproteins on the cholesterol bundle. This is how the cholesterol knows where to go. There are other variations on this combination of cholesterol and protein – mainly VLDL, or very low-density lipoprotein, and IDL, or intermediate density lipoprotein. These are made up of very little cholesterol, like HDL, but they have a high density of triglycerides- about 52%, or five times as much as LDL cholesterol. Their protein fraction is only 8%. They are constructed more like the chylomicrons (the suitcases in which fat is carried through intestinal walls) from which they are derived. The triglyceride portion can be made from sugar and starch – a fact that is lost on most advocates of a high carbohydrate diet! The levels of all these different cholesterols will fluctuate, depending on an individual's needs and the time of their last meal. They can be up-regulated to accommodate increased needs during times of chronic stress or growth.

LDL is the transporter that carries cholesterol, fats, and fat-soluble vitamins from our liver to our cells. Because it carries the cholesterol *to* cells and not away from them, it has been labelled 'bad cholesterol'. Once in the arteries cholesterol is released from its low-density lipoprotein shell into damaged tissue, where it accumulates, acting as an internal bandage on an artery sore. HDL cholesterol is the transporter that returns LDL cholesterol and fats from our diet and systemic circulation back to the liver, where they are removed from circulation and recycled. HDL is considered the 'good' cholesterol because it removes the LDL from the lining of artery walls, thereby limiting the amount of plaque build-up. All of this is indeed a good thing, and essential to managing ageing arteries that are constantly under attack as a result of lifestyle, environment and ageing itself. Atherosclerosis is primarily a disease of old age – a degenerative disease of the vascular endothelium, the single layer of cells on the inside of blood vessels, lymph vessels and heart vessels. It is these fragile arterial walls that benefit from the delivery of LDL cholesterol, which the body uses to patch them up if cells are damaged or break down.

Endothelial cell injury can also result from mechanical stress such as hypertension or a high level of *oxidized* LDL cholesterol, which is known to be toxic to endothelial cells. When the endothelial cell is injured there is an increased adherence of monocytes and T lymphocytes to the affected area. These are cells released as part of an immune response. Cytokines are the protein products of the monocytes and lymphocytes and they attract phagocytic cells to the sore spot. Phagocytes are cells that engulf foreign particles invading the body and then break them down. The cytokines, being the first on the scene, are the mediators of the atherogenic (plaque causing) process because they attract the phagocytes. The phagocytic cells surround the damaged LDL cholesterol, and then become engorged with lipids; in this state they are termed 'foam cells'. If they are numerous, the foam cells can infiltrate blood vessel walls, and as lipid accumulates, the lumen of the blood vessel involved is progressively closed off, or 'occluded'.

Cholesterol: cause or symptom?

This takes us back to Lands' assertion; what if shutting off the symptom isn't the best way to help the arterial wall heal? Yes, the oxidised LDL results in foam cells – but the LDL was sent there in the first place to deal with the damaged cells on the vessel wall. It is the oxidized LDL, rather than the 'native' or healthy LDL, which is the greater contributor to atherogenesis. Neutralizing the oxidation of the LDL with foods and supplements rich in antioxidants like vitamin E does not alter the function of LDL; it only slows down the decay of fatty acid chains that perpetuates phagocyte and foam cell proliferation.

But the HDL/ LDL classification, and the vilification of LDL cholesterol and its relationship with saturated fats, have become one more element in a distorted public understanding of fats and cholesterol. It has focused our attention onto a single, still controversial, blood component and away from a broader awareness of what constitutes a healthy lifestyle and diet. The obsession with cholesterol readings has given the public and their physicians a passive route to avoiding heart disease – simply substituting oils for hard fat. And it certainly would be a pretty easy way of avoiding a potentially fatal condition...if not for the fact that it isn't working.

Cholesterol's connection with cardiovascular disease is a result of its role in the protection of blood vessels, as described above. Contrary to widely held belief, lowering dietary cholesterol intake has only a temporary and minor affect on blood cholesterol. Compensatory mechanisms – basically an increase or decrease in the production and recycling of cholesterol – function to maintain the precarious endogenous cholesterol balance. Despite the body's ability to regulate cholesterol, there is a clear variation in how individuals respond to cholesterol in the diet. Some individuals respond weakly and others are strong responders; these are 'hyper' and 'hypo' cholesterol responders. Our mechanisms for cholesterol regulation will vary depending on the enzymes and receptors that we are born with.

There is also significant variability that has nothing to do with diet; an individual's health, or diet, or stress levels can lead them to respond very differently to dietary cholesterol at different times. Some of the mechanisms that account for differences in individual responses to dietary cholesterol include differences in the removal and excretion of cholesterol, differences in the formation and clearance of LDL cholesterol as regulated through specific receptors, and differences in the absorption or biosynthesis of cholesterol.

Possible causes of the contemporary increase in heart disease

These potential causes include: *deficiencies* of vitamin A, vitamin D, of antioxidants such as vitamin E and CoQ10, of ApoA/B (protein components of lipoproteins) and minerals. Other factors implicated in research results are: chronic stress; clotting; lipid oxidation; oxidized iron; hypothyroidism; hepatitis; kidney disease; gall bladder obstruction; viral and bacterial agents; oxidized omega 6; eicosanoid responses (inflammation), intake of trans fatty acids and pasteurised foods. And this does not include the changes in etiological frameworks and patterns of death reporting that seem to change rates of disease.

The potential for all these factors to cause heart disease has been established through the research of respected scientists. Many doctors and alternative practitioners are choosing to treat heart disease according to an etiology other than that of cholesterol levels and saturated fat intake. Heart disease is a very political ailment; other issues besides objective scientific analysis have had a profound effect on our understanding of the problem, and the first line of treatment is not necessarily the only or the best line of treatment. Heart disease is a compound disease with a diverse etiology, and diverse patterns of degeneration; it is not a condition with a single cause, so it is not a condition for which one solution will benefit all candidates. Read the theories of the dissenters before accepting at face value the standard, one-dimensional answers to a complex set of diseases and conditions.

16. William E.M. Lands Essential Fatty Acid Metabolism to Self-Healing Agents Healthful Lipids Oi-Ming Lai and Casimir C. Akoh AOCS Publishing 2005

CHAPTER 17

HOW OIL IS PROCESSED, WHAT HAPPENS WHEN WE COOK WITH IT

Where does oil come from?

Quality fat is a cornerstone of human nutritional health. And being aware of the overall quality of the oils available to us, especially the processing they undergo and the methods used to extract them, will help us to make truly informed choices.

Food fats and oils are derived from the oils in seed and animal sources. Animal fats are usually rendered from animal tissues using heat or steam to separate them from protein, which does not melt. Most of the rendered animal fats that you buy are extracted in approved rendering plants, which ensures their quality. Vegetable oils were traditionally extracted using cold or hot expression methods, but these have largely given way to solvent extraction because of the improved yield solvents can produce. The fats and oils obtained from rendering and extraction are referred to as 'crude' fats and oils, and will contain small amounts of other naturally occurring materials such as protein, free fatty acids, or phosphatides. These are usually removed with further processing. This processing may also eliminate some of the desirable elements of crude oils, such as the antioxidants vitamin E, carotene and lecithin – though technical advances have meant that all the desired natural antioxidants can be maintained, *if* the manufacturer chooses to do so.

Over the last century, the changes in the ways that we grow, extract and preserve all the foods that sustain us have been slow, sometimes almost imperceptible. But their cumulative effects have been profound. And this is especially true with fats and oils. For example, in Italy, oil pressing was traditionally a cottage industry, and each small village or large estate would have their own small oil press. Fresh oil used to be sold door to door, just like North Americans had milk and bread delivered to the house every morning.

The fatty acid profile of a fat or oil is not the only important factor in how it will influence our health. How an oil-yielding grain is grown and how the oil is extracted from the grain both affect the resulting product. Pesticides used on a grain crop will survive as pesticide residues in the oil extracted from the grain. If high temperatures are involved in the extraction, this will also affect the quality of the resulting oil. Solvents, light and oxygen all denature fatty acids, leading to further deterioration; the value of even the most healthful oils can be effectively negated by inappropriate extraction methods. Most prepared or partially prepared foods are made with inferior oils and fats. Even 'health food' products will often use less expensive and more stable modified fats.

Keep it in the fridge

One day I asked my husband to pick up a bottle of fresh flaxseed oil from our local high-end, high priced, fancy food market. When I got home, the opaque 300ml, $13.00 bottle was sitting on the counter. "Why isn't this in the fridge?" I asked. He furrowed his brow and said, "What do you mean? I bought it off the shelf. It wasn't in a refrigerator." Paolo went on to describe how all the oil products were displayed front and centre in the aisle, none of them in a fridge. A warning was clearly visible on the bottle, in capital letters; "KEEP REFRIGERATED". Oils rich in polyunsaturates must be kept refrigerated all the time; they are rich in omega 3 fatty acids, and these fats need to be kept consistently cool to minimize oxidation. Warmth will initiate breakdown; temperature change of any kind will do the same. Once a fat starts to break down it is essentially rancid and bad for our health. So here was a perfect example of one of nature's perfect foods being handled incorrectly – and becoming a health hazard as a consequence. Rancid flaxseed oil would cause a surge in free radical damage. Excessive free radicals require anti-oxidants for their neutralisation, and anti-oxidants are in high demand within our bodies; so any time we can conserve them by making a choice for stable fat rather than rancid fat we should do just that.

As with any food processing or refining, the extraction of oils from grains or nuts or seeds is something that can be done properly, with minimum damage to the food, or done rapidly and cheaply with no attention to the nutritional outcome. My bottle of flaxseed oil had been painstakingly extracted from organic flax seeds by a reputable company called Omega. It was expensive for a reason! But it had not been properly cared for all the way down the line to the point of sale, and as a result it was now worthless, perhaps even hazardous.

Human consumption of seed oils is a fairly recent development. It wasn't until the 1920s that the seed oil trade began to grow into a huge seed farming and oil extraction industry. The rapidly-growing volumes of seeds being processed led to the introduction of larger continuous screw presses, which replaced the smaller, cold temperature batch presses. Because they processed seeds continuously, these newer 'expeller' presses incidentally introduced heat into the process of extracting the oil. Heat had always been kept to a minimum in older methods, since it was understood to produce a product inferior in both taste and health properties. But even as an increasingly urbanised population was busy forgetting what was involved in growing and processing food, changes in technology and in the scale of farming and food production were having a direct, and largely unnoticed, effect on the quality of the oils available to consumers. Larger seed oil farms led to the use of pesticides. And the problem of potential residues in turn affected the ways in which oils were extracted. Secondary technologies for seed preparation, oil extraction, refinement, bleaching and deodorization were all developed to deal with problems such as residues, and oxidation during the initial extraction process. The emerging corporate food industry revolutionized the ways that seed oil was rendered, but there have been no net savings in the larger picture; the inferior oils they produce have simply externalised the costs, so that they are borne by our bodies and the health care system.

What the labels mean

If the debate about the health benefits of fats were based on the way they were refined rather than on the crude distinction between saturated and unsaturated, then the resulting government dietary recommendations would be very different. If consumers understood the nature and quality of the fats and oils they were buying, which are determined by the methods used to extract them, they would almost certainly be choosing different oils than they are now.

It can be very difficult to navigate through the maze of misinformation built in to the rules and conventions that determine how oils are labelled. The issue of labelling reminds me of the Dr. Seuss story 'The Sneetches'. Seems that the Star-Bellied Sneetches had a special label, and thought themselves special as a result. When that label was duplicated on other Sneetches who'd had no labels, it was impossible to tell who was an original Star-Bellied Sneetch. So much of our food supply is also "Sneetched", and as a result the labelling of foods can be a misleading business for the consumer. Most of us fall prey to it from time to time; we think we are purchasing one thing when in fact we are getting something entirely different.

Virgin oils

The best way to explain oil quality is to use the example of olive oil, since it is more familiar to us than the newer unsaturated fats. Everyone knows that 'virgin' olive oil is better than olive oil that doesn't come with this label. Virgin implies 'the first time', and virgin olive oil is made from the first pressing of the olives. As with every other aspect of the production of olive oil, this distinction is tightly regulated, in order to control and delineate quality. In the production of virgin olive oil, extraction temperature is controlled. Only unbruised, carefully handled olives can be used; once an olive is bruised its precious oils will start to denature. It is unfortunate that virgin olive oil is the only mass-marketed oil to have such well-defined protocols around its processing and raw materials. Other seed oils produced from virgin pressings are available in health food stores and in speciality grocery stores, but they are much less common. All oils marked with an authentic 'virgin' label must meet rigorous standards, and it is safe to assume that oil without this label has not been produced according to these standards.

Cold pressed oils

The degree of heat, light, and oxygen to which an oil is exposed will vary with different methods of processing and storage. Cold pressing is a process that creates no heat and involves minimal exposure to light and oxygen, thereby protecting an oil's nutritional quality and flavour. It does this by producing oil in single batches rather than continuously, in ways that allow for careful control of its exposure to the elements. You'll find cold-pressed oils in cans, green and brown glass bottles or black plastic bottles; clear bottles are never used for quality oil. A label that says 'virgin: cold pressed' assures you that extra care was taken producing the oil, and that the resulting oil isn't just better to eat; it's also better for you.

Mechanical expeller pressed oils

Seeds that are mechanically pressed to extract their oils are first cleaned and cooked for up to two hours. The cooking time depends on the toughness of the seed hull and how difficult it is to extract the oil from the seed inside. Cooking is basically a way to break food down, and the more cooking a seed undergoes the easier it will be to extract the oil. However, the more heat a seed is subjected to the more damage is done to the oils it contains, and the less healthful they become. It's the same principle we're all familiar with when it comes to steaming versus boiling vegetables. The more heat and water the vegetables are exposed to, the fewer nutrients they retain.

A mechanical expeller press for oil extraction is like a great big screw – a lot like the screw in old-fashioned manual meat grinders like the one Grandma Doolittle used to clamp to the edge of her kitchen table. The blades of a metal screw press down on the seeds, and along with this pressure comes heat, which increases as the blades press a continuous intake of seeds to produce a continuous flow of oil, leaving behind the 'oil cake', which is the fibre, skin, and protein of the seed. This by-product generally ends up in animal feed meal, or fertilizer. The greater the pressure on the seeds the greater the oil yields, but the higher the temperature as well, and the greater the damage done to this oil. Oil that is mechanically pressed with no restrictions concerning temperature, pressure or exposure to light or air can be sold in stores as 'unrefined oil'. It is implied that unrefined' equals wholesome, but the exposure to heat and oxygen inherent in the expeller process means that mechanical 'expeller pressed oil' has been subject to oxidation, vitamin E deterioration, and free radical damage. This labelling is fundamentally misleading. These oils have been touted as inherently health-enhancing foods, but they clearly have the potential to cause harm.

I am privy to the eating habits of my clients and lecture attendees, and I have discovered that many people do not recognize the smell of rancid frying oil. When you walk past a 'greasy spoon' restaurant, the odour of oil cooked many times without being changed is offensive, isn't it? Remember that smell, and see if you can smell it on your dinner; that is the smell of poor quality oil. You can taste it as well; and you can taste *good* oil as surely as you can taste bad oil.

Solvent extraction

The raw material of solvent extraction is the seed meal produced by mechanical pressing; seeds are first pressed mechanically, and then a chemical solvent such as heptane (also available commercially as rubber cement solvent and camping stove fuel!) or hexane (defined as a hazardous air pollutant by the EPA!) is introduced to the remaining seed cake. The solvent, combined with heat and agitation, ensures the extraction of virtually all of the remaining oil in the seed meal. Solvent-extracted oils and expeller pressed oils can be blended together and sold as 'unrefined' – and commonly are.

Solvent extracted oils go on to be deodorized to remove the chemical odour of the heptane, degummed, and refined. My mother used to use these oils from time to time for frying, and she probably still does when I'm not around. I once asked her why she used them, and she replied, "Well Melissa," (when she uses my full name I know she is perturbed by my query), "It doesn't burn, you know." Of course it doesn't burn, look what it has already been through; heat extraction at 325 degrees or more, hexane, bleaching, and degumming, which removes all the life enhancing phospholipids. This is not a viable food product, and there is no good reason to eat solvent extracted refined oils.

Always choose virgin pressed oils, and store them according to the instructions! True virgin oils will come in opaque glass or plastic bottles. Clear glass represents a 'clear' oversight when it comes to the procedures necessary to preserve oil quality. Always put the cap back on your oil; don't leave it exposed to air. Unrefined, refined and mechanically pressed oils are less healthy than virgin oils. Use them only for stovetop frying, or avoid them completely.

And for Lord's sake stop judging the healthfulness of a fat solely on the basis of its status as saturated or unsaturated! The story of the procedures inflicted on the saturated fats in palm, coconut, and milk is equally appalling. But because saturated fats are more stable, and suffer less damage from exposure to heat, pressure and air, they are better able to survive the extraction process intact and relatively healthful. This means that a saturated fat's fatty acid profile is passed on to the consumer in a relatively natural and unchanged form.

'Fixing' solvent-extracted oil

The degraded quality of solvent extracted oil, and the market expectation (created by food producers) that oil should be pristine, transparent, odourless and non-smoking, means that commercial oils are subjected to several more processes before they are bottled and sent on their way.

Degumming: This is done to remove phospholipid compounds from oils prior to refining. (Remember phospholipids are essential for brain function.) The unrefined oil is treated with a limited amount of water to hydrate the phospholipids and make them separable. Soy is the most commonly degummed oil; the removed phospholipids are processed further and sold separately as lecithin, which is a known cholesterol emulsifier. Advances in degumming include using a combination of sodium hydroxide and citric acid mixed with water and enzymes to create a stable emulsion. The emulsion allows the enzymes to react with the phospholipids, making them water-soluble and easier to remove from the oil. The oil yield with enzyme degumming is higher than traditional methods, and the recovered phospholipids are processed further to yield a variety of lecithin products.

Bleaching: This refers to any process used to remove colour-producing substances, along with other trace particles, from oil. This includes the colour producing substances chlorophyll and beta carotene. The most common method of bleaching involves the absorption of impurities by a material such as acid-activated bleaching earth or clay (bentonite). Bentonite consists primarily of hydrated aluminium silicate. If there are any essential fatty acids in the oil, bleaching can result in the production of toxic peroxides and conjugated fatty acids.

Deodorization: This is a vacuum steam distillation process; steam is sucked through oil to remove volitile trace constituents that can give rise to undesirable flavours, colours, and odours. It's usually done after the degumming and bleaching processes. Deodorizing does not have a significant negative effect on all oils, but it can produce small amounts of trans fatty acids in those with a high proportion of unsaturated fatty acids.

Fractionation/ winterization: Fractionation is a general term for the separation of the components in a liquid. It can involve distillation, solvents, or the manipulation of temperature – though distillation obviously doesn't work all that well with oil. Winterization is a specific process in which material is crystallized by cooling, and removed from the oil by filtration, all to avoid oil becoming cloudy at cooler temperatures. (Oh now that would be just awful wouldn't it.)

Interesterification: This restructures the original fatty acid line-up along the glycerol molecule to produce speciality fats with particular melting curves desired by food producers. Chemical interesterification is a process catalysed by sodium methoxide. When the process is complete the catalyst is neutralized and the rearranged product is washed, bleached and deodorized to give it its final desired characteristics. Interestification can also be achieved with enzymes.

Esterification: Fatty acids are usually present in nature in the form of esters, especially esters of glycerol They are further digested by the body into esters of di-glycerides and mono-glycerides. Esterification is basically the opposite process; an alcohol is reacted with a fatty acid to form an ester of mono or diglycerides. This process yields useful food ingredients that emulsify in food production.

Read the labels when you buy processed foods that contain fats. You will start to become aware of the industrial realities behind the reassuring images of 'heart-friendly' vegetable oils, and the significance of terms like 'hydrogenated', or the more obscure but equally significant 'modified'. *Minimizing* our consumption of fats that have been subjected to these refining processes is always going to be the best way to *maximise* the health benefits of the fats and oils in our diet. The fresher and more natural your diet, the less modified fat and oil you will be ingesting, and the better your chances of achieving a healthy dietary balance of fatty acids.

Hydrogenation

Trans fatty acids have had their day in the courts, and most consumers are now aware of the negative impact these unnaturally deformed fats can have on our health. The biochemistry of hydrogenation was covered in the margarine section, but a quick review can't hurt. Hydrogenation takes unsaturated liquid oils like cotton seed, canola, or mixed vegetable oil as its starting product. A nickel catalyst is pumped into the oil under high heat and pressure, causing the hydrogen atoms of the oils to flip to the opposite sides of their fatty acid chains. Their cis configuration changes to a trans configuration, making the oil progressively more solid. "Cis" means the hydrogen atoms are on the same side of the fatty acid chain, which makes the fatty acid fluid because the hydrogens bend and twist in unison. The hydrogen atoms on opposite sides of the "trans" fatty acid create a more rigid structure, preventing the unsaturated fatty acid from moving so freely. Technically, hydrogenated oils are unsaturated; but biochemically they behave like super long chain saturated fats. Ultimately, this is *not* a good thing for cellular metabolism.

The solid fat that results from the hydrogenation process is spreadable – it mimics the consistency of room temperature butter. For a long time margarine was believed by most health practitioners to be superior to butter or coconut oil, and most physicians insisted on hydrogenated margarines for heart patients, or anyone with a keen interest in health. However, as the biochemistry of these substances became more widely known, and as scientists like Dr. Mary Enig carried out new lipid hydrogenation research, it became increasingly clear that hydrogenated fats were interfering with cellular metabolism and wreaking havoc on cell receptors for insulin, as well as causing people's blood lipid profiles to rise

above normal balanced levels. And hydrogenation is not the only negative attribute of liquid oils turned into spreadable margarines. The oils
used for margarines are heavily processed, under extreme heat and pressure, and rich in the wrong sorts of residues – residues from industrial
processes, not from the natural product that might have been. In short:
foods created by hydrogenation are invariably harmful, and should be
avoided like botulism and mad dogs.

CHAPTER 18

FATS IN A NUTSHELL

Fats in a nutshell

You could look at the messages that this book has tried to get across in two different lights. The first would emphasise the central, narrowly scientific concerns of the book: We are eating too much omega 6-rich vegetable oil, which is damaging our health by overstimulating our pro-inflammatory responses and contributing to a host of problems, from arthritis to allergies to heart disease to cancer. On the other hand, our diets are seriously deficient in omega 3, in part because we no longer eat foods that contain it, and in part because those omega 6 fatty acids compete with omega 3 for the other nutritional co-factors that enable our bodies to make use of them. Saturated fat is a useful and indeed a necessary part of the human diet, and its molecular stability makes it a far more healthful choice for virtually any foods that involve cooking. Unsaturated fats of all kinds, but especially those same omega 6- rich vegetable oils, are subjecting our bodies to a burden of oxidation that both causes damage in its own right and makes severe demands on our reserves of antioxidants, which really have better things to do. Some of us should be eating less fat and oil, and some of us should be eating more; but almost all of us should be eating a far greater *variety* of fats and oils.

The second light would focus on a set of interconnected common sense ideas: All fats can contribute to human health, if they are eaten in the appropriate amounts and proportions, and providing they come from natural sources and have been treated well – fats have long memories, and will almost always take any violence done to *them* out on *us*. You could broaden this message and say that eating in a way that reflects and respects the habits embedded in traditional diets around the world is the best and easiest way to find your way back to nutritional health. The human spirit may be racing towards the future on the wings of technology, but our bodies remain stubbornly rooted in nature, and need natural foods to flourish. Blaming butter, beef and palm oil for health problems that have actually been caused by industrial-scale meddling with the food we inescapably need is to some extent a way of blaming *people*, and disarming them in the face of these attempts to reshape our diets according to the interests of corporations and the science they make such careless use of. This might seem like a peculiar message from a book that has involved so much biochemistry – but I'd justify it by suggesting that after a century of delusion, lost in its infatuation with the marvels of mass production and mass communication, the science of nutrition is in many ways only now catching up with the common sense inherent in these traditional diets, and only now becoming a true friend of health rather than a false one. If I were feeling more pessimistic I would say that science is a tool that can be used for good or ill – just like the guy in the white hat and the guy in the black hat in that old cowboy movie both have guns.

Oils for health

Fats are vital to human health, and maintaining a balance between saturated fats, monounsaturated fats and essential omega fats is an important step to a healthy metabolism, and to good overall health. Fats help *stimulate* our metabolisms and enhance muscle repair. Consuming fat can actually *decrease* body fat storage. Essential fats make cells more sensitive to insulin, helping them metabolise sugar better. Fats transport vital nutrients and the fat-soluble vitamins A, D, E, and K. Fat is essential to the health of our heart, lungs, bones, gonads, endocrine system and brains. Saturated fat helps us assimilate calcium.

Trans fatty acids do exist in nature, and our bodies can metabolise them, but *artificial* trans fatty acids are detrimental to human health and should be eliminated from our diet altogether. Fried foods, though not health enhancing, are tolerated by the body. The high heat of frying denatures fats and creates free radical damage and trans isomers. Free radicals damage our cellular DNA, the first step in the development of many diseases. A diet rich in foods that provide us with anti-oxidants is a good defence against the damage that bad fats can inflict. To minimize the detrimental affects of frying, it's best to use stable saturated fats such as palm oil, coconut oil, beef tallow and lard.

Unsaturated fats, such as those in safflower, canola, sunflower and soy oils, do have health benefits – but these are largely lost with the high temperatures and uncontrolled exposure to air and light involved in the most common extraction processes. With monounsaturated fats, only virgin pressings should be used, and never for high heat cooking.

Nature takes care of endogenous fat ratios – animals' as well as ours – and the meat of an animal fed a healthy diet will contain a healthy, balanced critical ratio of fats. Our bodies are equipped to deal with highly saturated animal fat which contains a balanced critical ratio; they will convert any excess fatty acids to more useful forms of fat. Like all other foods, fat can be harmful, as when certain fats are eaten out of balance with others, or when too many processed fats, like trans fats or refined fats, take the place of naturally stable fats like coconut oil, palm oil, or butter, or when we simply eat too much fat. Nothing in this book should be read as inviting people to eat all the fat they can. That's what the food industry is doing, in a way, by producing its mountains of 'good for us' foods.

It's important to remember that these fat-related truths have to be understood in the context of the rest of the foods in your diet; no food exercises its effects, for good or ill, in isolation from all the other nutrients the body takes in. So in order to understand the effects of fats on our health we need to look at their synergistic interaction with everything else we eat. Just because a food such as milk or meat contains a "saturated" fat, which on its own is "hypercholesterolemic" (cholesterol raising) should not imply that it will raise one's cholesterol levels – this is something determined by the *whole* diet. Simply isolating foods and nutrients into 'good' and 'bad' categories is a flawed approach to evaluating a specific food's effect on health.

It's up to us

Each of us must decide our own level of commitment to ensuring the quality and variety of the fats in our diet, and to preparing foods using the types of oil that meet our nutritional needs and health expectations. Whatever our level of commitment, our food choices should take account of the quality of food, including its freshness and ripeness, whether it was grown with or without pesticides, and how it has been processed and prepared. The quality and origin of a food and its ingredients are just as important as its protein, carbohydrate and fat content.

In our household we use unrefined flaxseed oil on salads, and occasionally it is used as a dietary supplement. Butter is used on steamed vegetables and bread, and in baking. We use olive oil for quick cooking on top of the stove, for dipping bread, and with tomatoes. Grape seed oil and coconut oil are used for higher temperature cooking. When he is feeling particularly hedonistic, my husband will fry potatoes in unrefined vegetable oil. (The higher the oleic acid/ omega 9 content of a vegetable oil, relative to its omega 6 content, the more stable it will be.) We do not use refined oils in our home! However when visiting mothers, or friends, or eating at the local diner, I am sure we are getting a dose of margarine, solvent extracted vegetable oil or shortening. You can't be healthy every waking minute. Develop guidelines for the types of fats that suit your lifestyle and health concerns, and try making improvements one step at a time. Worrying too much about how an oil was refined will do as much harm to your arteries as the wrong food ever could! I suggest changing the variety of fat in your diet as gradually as is necessary in order to stay relaxed with the process. Enjoy the new flavours – and enjoy the knowledge that you're bestowing goodness and health on yourself and your family.

So how do we make all these changes? The first step is easy; if food is natural, unrefined and unprocessed it is generally going to be healthy, so feel free to eat it. The second step is almost as easy: eat a sensible balance of foods, and don't be led astray by official advice, or by media or industry 'advice' that tries to sound official for its own purposes. The past decade has seen a constant parade of senseless dietary panics: carrots have been vilified for having more sugar in them than broccoli, and baked potatoes for being too starchy compared to boiled ones. This obsessive hyper-management of good foods versus bad is futile (especially when it comes to vegetables and fruits!). It can make meal times unbearable, and far more complicated than if we listened just a bit more closely to our primal instincts. Eat fresh, embrace variety, avoid cans and boxes, eat local where possible, and remember that you are a part of nature, and it is a part of you. Your Grandma knew this too!

CHAPTER 19

PUTTING IT ALL TOGETHER: RECIPES, PRACTICAL TIPS FOR PLANNING MEALS, AND SUGGESTIONS FOR EASY-TO-FOLLOW PATTERNS OF EATING

How do you go about turning a book full of information into a change in your lifestyle? It shouldn't be a complicated process; take it slowly and change things one step at a time. I've tried to offer advice throughout the book. If some of it stands out in your memory, perhaps it indicates a good place to start. This chapter gives some more ideas that I've found helpful over the years, because they work, and because the lifestyle changes they represent are easy, and the effects are positive. And because the recipes are tasty!

Proper nutrition is far easier than arranging for pre-packaged food from a diet clinic or food delivery service. Eating well certainly does not have to involve shopping in a health food store or eating foods that are not commonly available. Good food can be fast food too. Preparing and cooking fish is a 12 minute process – less time than it takes to make a package of Sloppy Joes.

Watch the portions. Good wholesome food does not make you fat; *too much food* makes you fat. Over the past 23 years I've been in the nutrition business, the people I've had the opportunity to help lose weight did not originally get fat from eating too much steak and eggs and butter. They did it from eating foods they binged on, eating outside of regular meal times and eating foods that were devoid of nutrition – like chips, and pastries. One fellow even gained weight while training for a marathon, from sucking back supplemental gel packs every 40 minutes while he was running! Stick to balanced meals and avoid erratic meal patterns at all costs. Proper nutrition will fuel all of your activities, and all your working life challenges.

Coconut is an excellent source of healthy saturated fats, and I've featured it a bit in the recipes and advice that follows. This is partly because it's such an easy way to introduce saturated fat into your diet, and also because I find a lot of people don't have any idea how to cook with coconut milk, meat or oil. But once you start experimenting with these delightful foods you will not want to go a day without them.

Coconut oil can be used in baking or for stop top sautéing. Always buy organic, high quality coconut oil where possible. It should be in an opaque jar or bottle, and be odourless and tasteless. *Creamed coconut* can be found in the refrigerated section of many grocery stores, and of course in Indian and Asian markets. It is made from the finely chopped meat of the coconut, and all the valuable oils are still in it. The hard white blocks can be melted in broths, soups, sauces and curries.

Canned, whole *coconut milk* is the product we use most often at home. It is now widely available in most grocery stores in the canned food section. It's best to buy the organic version, as the regular version is processed with sulfites, which can cause allergic reactions. Never buy the 'lite' version – it's the fat that you want! Add coconut milk to broth, soups, sauces, curries, smoothies or any concoction you make in your blender. Add it to rice and bean dishes as well. *Desiccated coconut* is the 'meat' of the coconut. The unsweetened version is the best; it can be used on top of desserts, mixed into yoghurt and added to favourite cookie recipes. Read the label; sulfites are often used here as well, so beware.

Suggested meal plans

Breakfast

Option 1: Breakfast to Go or To Stay

This is a breakfast that I recommend to many clients, and eat several times a week myself. A fat-rich meal like this maintains satiety and helps you make it to lunch without feeling hungry. It's Andy Pringle's least favourite:

2 tablespoons full fat coconut milk

¾ cup full fat kefir *or*

2 tablespoons full fat yoghurt

½ cup berries of your choice

1 full tablespoon of each of the following – sunflower seeds, ground flaxseeds, hemp seeds or protein powder, pumpkin seeds and walnuts

2-4 tablespoons of rolled oats, either raw or pre-soaked in water the night before.

This fits nicely into a small container to eat on the go. Or have it at home with your fresh-brewed coffee and cream – but do try to forgo the sugar in that coffee.

Option 2: Breakfast Smoothie To Go

This is definitely a breakfast for on the go. Feel free to mix and match the ingredients. It travels well but tastes best cool. If you choose to add the protein isolate supplement recall that this *needs* fat for its protein to be assimilated, so don't skimp on the fat content.

In a blender add the following ingredients:

1 frozen banana

3-6 ice cubes

3 tablespoons coconut milk

1 scoop of protein isolate (I prefer ENG organic plain whey protein)

Enough buttermilk for the consistency that you prefer.

Water if you prefer your smoothie a bit less thick

Mix all the ingredients at high speed. Add water or buttermilk to suit your taste and texture preferences. Depending on the protein supplement that you choose this can be a very high protein breakfast – it will average about 30 grams of protein. Remember you'll need plenty of fat to aid the assimilation of the protein. Feel free to add any blue-green algae supplement to increase the antioxidant concentration.

Option 3: Oatmeal Winter Breakfast

I like this breakfast in the cold winter months. I find that with the cold weather and the dark mornings I feel much more contented with a bit of a heavier feeling in my gut. To make oatmeal efficiently in the morning I mix the proper amount of oats with the proper ratio of water the night before, and put the mixture in the fridge. During the night the oats soak up the water and the starch content in the oats starts to break down. This is a 'slow cook' version of preparing oatmeal; in the morning the oats are essentially 'cooked.' If you prefer them warmed up just stir the pot of oats with a little added water over a medium heat for a minute or two. Add your important fats and a bit of fruit for fibre.

Suggested Toppings for Oatmeal Breakfast:
    2-3 tablespoons of coconut milk
    Some shredded apple
    Dash of cinnamon
    3-4 tablespoons each of chopped almonds and flax seeds
    *Un*homogenized milk to taste
    If you need to have a bit more sweetness add a bit of sugar or honey

(Some Coconut-free Breakfast Options)

Option 4: Eggs
    2 poached eggs on top of 1 slice of generously buttered spelt toast
    Topped with ¼ cup of steamed spinach and a slice of Asiago cheese

(I often have this breakfast for a lunchtime meal, and the spinach is often leftover from dinner the night before with a clove or two of garlic)
    This is by far my favourite breakfast.

Breakfast Option 5: Toast and Peanut Butter
    1 slice spelt toast and peanut butter. (That was easy!)

Each slice of spelt toast has 9 grams of protein and 15 grams of carbohydrates. The peanut butter tops up the protein and fat content and will stick to your ribs. When I make this breakfast it is usually in the winter after a couple of morning clients. I spread butter on the toast before the peanut butter – it makes it much saltier, and great with a burning hot coffee. I will add a crunchy fruit to get my fibre quotient up.

Breakfast Option 6: Bacon and Eggs
    Poached or scrambled eggs (scrambled gives you an opportunity to
        mix the eggs with whole milk before cooking)
    2 slices of bacon
    Sliced tomato with basil and olive oil
    1 slice of toast with butter

In a rush? Eggs can be eaten cold! Cooked up a day or two in advance and stored in a glass container scrambled eggs and room temperature bacon make a fine start to the morning if time is of the essence.

Breakfast Option 7: Salmon on Toast
    1 slice of toasted spelt or pita
    3-4 oz of smoked salmon
    Capers, lemon, and 2 tablespoons of full fat quark

Quark is a natural product – pressed and slightly creamed cheese. It is high in probiotics, protein and quality fats. Find it in the dairy section of modern grocery stores. Quark was served at the Plaza Hotel in New York the last time I was there. It is becoming ubiquitous and displacing commercial cream cheese.

Lunch
Lunch Option 1: Green Salad with Chicken and Potatoes
    2 cups of mixed greens, including arugula, spinach, romaine lettuce....
    3 tablespoons of blue cheese
    Sliced tomato, cucumber, onion
    ¼ cup steamed baby potatoes
    ¼ cup cold chicken strips
    Dress with olive oil, lemon, salt and pepper or flaxseed oil with hot pepper. (You can buy flaxseed oil like this.) This salad would serve two if you added a slice of spelt bread.

Lunch Option 2: Stuffed Baked Potato

Small to medium baked potato, stuffed with...

½ cup of tuna mixed with mayonnaise, onion, capers, salt and pepper. Can be topped with ½ tablespoon of sour cream and chives.

This is a portable lunch if you use a recyclable container to pack it in. The potatoes can be cooked ahead of time and the skins left on.

Lunch Option 3: Leftovers (!)

Leftovers from your dinner. Put them in a container, freshen up the dressings and toppings and be off for the day.

Lunch Option 4: A Nice Restaurant

Eating in a restaurant? Choose a protein-centred meal and forgo the sandwich. Get your carbohydrates from the vegetables and fruit. Save the bread for an at-home meal when you can control the quality of the flour that you are eating. After a hard workout I like to have a hamburger. Check out the neighbourhood around where you work for restaurants that serve fresh foods, and that keep the meal focused on vegetables and proteins rather than on starchy foods that fill you up but leave out those quality, satisfying fats.

Burger Lunch:

A 6-8 oz sirloin burger on top of a plate of mixed vegetables, topped with cheese and pickles – plus a side salad. I will often buy a Voortman's cookie on the way back to the office (they're made with palm oil or butter) and have it with a tea once I am at my desk, before hitting the gym floor.

Bistro Lunch:

At my favourite Italian bistro I usually opt for the fish special, which is served with plenty of steamed and dressed vegetables. For dessert I'll have a decaffeinated cappuccino made with whole milk. My husband calls this 'mange-cake' eating, as Italians only have cappuccino for breakfast and decaffeinated coffee is a sacrilege. If I'm with my friend, mentor and colleague Carol we have wine. Those lunches with a glass of wine can be very productive indeed!

Now on to Dinner

Your dinner should fill the gap left by whatever you missed at lunch and breakfast time. If I've had the burger for lunch I would likely want fish for dinner. The vegetables that you prepare for dinner can be used the next day for lunches. Paolo takes vegetables that as a Canadian I can only imagine being eaten warm, and serves them cold. He'll take things like string beans or broccoli, steam them, and then put in the fridge, to be dressed later in olive or sesame oil, garlic, lemon, salt and pepper and served with the meal. The leftovers are packed up for my lunch the next day. The longer they marinate the better they taste.

Dinner should never have to be ascetic or boring. Stay away from packaged foods – if your time is limited, just keep it simple, as in the suggestions below. Basically, dinner should be one third protein, one third carbohydrate, and one third fat – including the fat you add to your foods *and* the fat in the protein. The hardest part of eating well for people who work is often the shopping. Maybe grocery delivery is an option, or sharing the load with others.

Dinner Option 1: Fish
    Whole grilled fish with lemon
    Green salad with dressing
    ½ to 1 cup pasta primavera with olive oil dressing
    1 glass of red wine
    1 oz old cheese

Dinner Option 2: Beef
    Beef Bourguignon
    Side salad
    1 slice of sour dough rye bread
    1 glass of wine

Dinner Option 3:Eggplant Parmesan
   Chicken or veal consume
   6 inch serving of Eggplant Parmesan
   Salad with dressing
   1 glass wine

Dinner Option 4: Stir Fry
   Stir-fry.....
   1-2 cups of cubed vegetables in sesame oil and chicken stock, with
   ¼ cup of coconut milk
   6 oz of cubed chicken per person
   serve with
   ½ - 1 cup brown rice per person
   1 glass wine

Stocks

Beef, veal, chicken and fish stocks are favourite treats year-round; Paolo makes gallons of stock and we give it away to clients in big one-litre mason jars. It's a universal favourite, and they always get more as long as the jars are returned. If anyone is overlooked when we hand out the stock, they always let us know that they are waiting with anticipation for the next batch. The potential nutritional contribution of soup stocks is overlooked nowadays, with our rushed, on-the-go mentality. But stock is a regular meal starter in our home. Once you find out just how easy it is to make, and feel the benefits it bestows, you'll want to make it a regular part of your diet.

Stocks are extremely nutritious because they contain the minerals of the bone, cartilage and marrow. Paolo always adds wine while the pot of bones is simmering. This, we later learned, helps to draw the minerals calcium, magnesium and potassium out of the bones and into the broth. My Grandma didn't know this, but she added wine vinegar to her stock, which accomplishes the same thing. Most cooked foods repel water, making them harder to digest. But the gelatin in stock attracts liquids to the gut, so a bowl of broth at the start of a meal makes for better digestion and a more complete assimilation of nutrients. There is an abundance of amino acids (the building blocks of proteins) in bones, and in broth – notably arginine, proline and glycine. These help the body make better use of the other amino acids in the diet, especially those from non-meat sources. Proteins are never absorbed directly by the body; they're always broken down into amino acids in the gut, and then put back together as needed, with specific amino acids for specific purposes. (We'll leave all that for another book!) Making stock from soup bones helps make sure nothing is wasted, the least we can do for the animals we eat, and our bodies benefit because stock helps us achieve a complete and balanced diet.

Chicken Stock
   1 free-range chicken, about 2 pounds
   4 litres of filtered water
   1 large onion, diced
   2 large carrots, sliced
   3-6 stocks of celery, sliced
   ½ cup red wine

If you can find it, the whole chicken, with the head on, can be used. Waste not, want not! Cut the chicken into several pieces and place these in a large stainless steel pot with the water and wine (or vinegar!). Let stand for 30 minutes, then slowly bring to a boil. Simmer on low heat for 6 hours, removing the scum that collects on the top of the water. If you want a more concentrated stock that can be stored more easily, simmer it longer – so that the excess water boils off. This water can be added back to the stock when you are ready to use it again.

Remove the stock from the heat and fish out the chicken pieces with a slotted spoon. While the stock is still hot add a bunch of parsley sprigs. The chicken meat that is removed can be used for other meals such as chicken salads or curries.

You are done. The stock can be separated into 1 or ½ litre jars and stored for several months in the freezer, or several weeks in the fridge. If you're storing in the freezer, it's a good idea to use a non leaching plastic container.

Veal Broth

Pour 4-6 litres of room temperature, filtered water into a large cauldron. Add:

2 pounds of veal shank
2-3 carrots in large pieces
4-5 stalks chopped celery
½ onion
½ ball of fennel chopped
Whole stem parsley
1 medium tomato cut into quarters
Fresh basil leaves
Salt and pepper

Bring to a boil – this will take about 45 minutes to an hour.

Skim the fat after broth has boiled briefly. Add seasoning as needed, and ½ cup of red wine or wine vinegar, then let it simmer for one hour.

Take out the meat and bones and vegetables, and put in separate container. Pour the soup mix through a strainer lined with cheesecloth. If it's not tasty enough you can reduce it further over low heat.

The vegetables can be used for minestrone soup. The veal can served as a side dish with pickled vegetables such as beets, artichokes, mushrooms or carrots, or olives. This is *sottaceto,* which means 'under vinegar', and is very good for digestion. Some of the veal shank can be shredded into the broth. Add rice or egg to make broth more substantial.

You can substitute four pounds of soup bones (short ribs or beef shank crosscuts) for the meat. Get them from the butcher and simmer for several hours instead of one.

After-Dinner Desserts

Chocolate Yum-yums:

This is a supremely easy refrigerator cookie recipe. I have been making these since I was a young teenager experimenting in the kitchen, and I have finally mastered them. I once used salt in place of sugar and my brother hasn't eaten my cookies since. Too bad for him; I can make really tasty cookies now.

1 cup butter
3 tablespoons cocoa
1 dark chocolate bar, or semi-sweet baking chocolate
1 cup sugar
2 cups of desiccated coconut
Splash of vanilla
Milk, if required, to adjust the consistency of the paste

Melt the chocolate and butter over a double saucepan. When they have blended, remove them from the heat and mix in the coconut, vanilla and sugar. A paste-like consistency will develop and the mix should stick together easily.

If the mixture gets too thick, add in milk by the tablespoon to return the mixture to a sticky but manageable consistency.

Drop by spoonfuls on to a waxed paper cookies sheet. Refrigerate for a couple of hours. Done.

Coconut Pie Crust:

This adds a whole new dimension to pie. Easy to do and it can be stored if you make more than one at a time. You can use coarsely shredded coconut – simply chop it more finely in a food processor to get the right consistency.

½ cup melted butter
2 cups finely chopped coconut.

Mix the melted butter in a bowl then add the coconut and mix well. Press into a 9 inch pie plate and bake at 300 degrees for 30 minutes. Allow to cool at room temperature before adding in the filling.

Apple Pie Filling
> 8-10 medium tart apples, peeled, cored and cut into medium sized
> chucks
> 2 tablespoons arrowroot powder
> 2 tablespoons sucanat (unrefined cane sugar – highly nutritious)
> Grated lemon rind
> 1 teaspoon cinnamon

Fill the pie crust with the apple chunks. Mix the arrowroot, sucanat, cinnamon and lemon peel and sprinkle the mixture over the apples. With any remaining coconut crust cover the top of the pie with a lattice. Bake at 375 degrees for 45 minutes or until the filling bubbles. Cool before serving.

Dessert Mousse for Six
> 6 egg yolks at room temperature
> ½ cup honey or maple syrup
> Grated rind of 2 lemons
> Juice of 2 lemons
> 6 egg whites at room temperature
> Pinch of sea salt
> ½ cup heavy non-pasteurized cream well chilled

Place the egg yolks, honey or syrup, lemon rind and lemon juice in the top of a double broiler over simmering water. Whisk constantly for about 10 minutes until the mixture thickens. Remove and chill in the fridge for about ½ hour. Beat cream until still. In a separate bowl, beat the egg whites with salt until still. Fold the lemon mixture into the cream and then the egg whites into the resulting mixture. Spoon into individual parfait glasses and chill well before serving. Can be garnished with fresh mint.

The Famous Two Day Rotation Diet

Throughout my years as a practitioner I have found that clients often struggle with diets because the foods they are eating too much of, and feel an addiction to, are the very foods that are negatively impacting their metabolism, in any number of ways. The offending food isn't necessary eaten in excessive amounts, but it is eaten regularly. I use the two day rotation diet as a simple means of isolating the foods that cause cravings, and as a way to help up-regulate the metabolism. Most people feel cleansed and energized after they've done a rotation diet perfectly for the full two days. After the two day process, I recommend that people go back to their normal diet; the offending foods are usually easily recognizable, and have less attraction for people. I often see that addictions to diet pop, heavy starchy lunches, sugary drinks and mid-day coffee have abetted. Many people look forward to the two day diets, and eventually do not stray far from the diet in their regular eating patterns.

You will notice a common theme in the rotation diets, one of which is a lack of flour based foods. Flour based meals, or meals with most of the calories in the form of flour. are the norm in our society. Because of the way flour is digested, and the ways it affects the assimilation of other nutrients, its removal from the diet leaves many people feeling more focused, with better energy. The rotation diet also encourages regular meal patterning. The strict meal times help re-establish the discipline of eating on a regular basis. This helps to moderate the tendency to overeat, and also lets the body recognize feelings of satiety. The cycle of hunger and feeding can be re-established much more easily. Digestive enzymes will be ready and waiting for you to eat.

I encourage you to try out a rotation diet. Choose the one that best suits your needs. The title and the brief description of each diet will give you some idea of the objective of the diet, and for whom it is ideally suited. Then go back to your regular eating – hopefully with more awareness of how you are feeling and what your body is asking you to eat.

Weekly Rotation Diet

Breakfast
    2 poached eggs
    1 slice 7 grain organic toast (no wheat) with butter
    Fruit of choice

Lunch
> 2 cups lentil soup, I slice toasted 7 grain organic bread (no wheat)
> Mixed salad with peppers, green onion, celery, with olive oil and
> > garlic

Dinner
> ½ glass wine
> 4-6 oz steak
> 2-3 cups steamed asparagus and broccoli with butter and garlic
> If hungry have more vegetables dressed with butter
> (Fiber – 45 grams, protein 60-65 grams)

Weight Loss Rotation Diet with Cardio

Day 1
> AM: Cardio before any food intake one hour intervals or fartlek. Before cardio have ½ cup hot black coffee no milk or cream. After cardio take 30-45 minutes to clean up before eating anything. Have water with lemon right away.

Breakfast
> 2 poached eggs,
> 1-2 sliced tomatoes with oil and salt and pepper,
> 3 strips of bacon

Lunch
> 4-6 oz burger, dressed with onion, mustard but no condiments
> > with sugar.
> Selection of green vegetables to your heart's content.
> After meal have peppermint tea, or ginger, or lemon or fennel tea.

Dinner
> 1 cup pasta dressed in tomato, meat or tuna sauce
> 1 glass of red wine
> Salad dressed in oil and vinegar

Day 2

AM: Run after ½ cup black coffee 30 minutes. After run take 30-45 minutes before breakfast

Breakfast
    ¼ cup oats with ½ cup full-fat kefir
    2 tablespoons each of walnuts, flax, coconut (no sulfites) sunflower
        seeds, pumpkin   seeds

Lunch
    4 oz tuna mixed with oil
    1 slice wheat-free bread
    Side salad as large as you like, and full of non-cruciferous vegetables
    dressed in flaxseed oil.

Dinner
    1 whey protein shake
    2-3 cups broccolini dressed in butter and garlic
    No wine – just go to bed.

Grandma's Rotation Diet

Breakfast, 7:00 – 8:30 am
    2 poached eggs
    3 oz tomato or vegetable juice
    2 slices bacon
    1 slice of whole grain toast and butter
    ½ cup mixed chopped fruit
    Coffee with cream

Lunch, 12:00 – 1:00 pm
    4-6 oz leftover meat or chicken
    ½ cup cold potato salad
    1 large apple
    Cup of tea with honey

Dinner, between 5:30 – 7:00 pm
    1 bowl of veal consume
    6 oz liver with onions
    1 full cup of string beans, corn, carrot medley
    3 tablespoons of fermented vegetables, onions, garlic, cucumbers,
        cabbage

Dessert
    3 tablespoons *crème fraîche* with 1 cup of fruit in season
    Tea and milk

GLOSSARY

Adipose tissue: Another term for fat deposits, though most adipose tissue is only about 80% fat, with the rest being tissues for servicing or utilising the deposits. Specific locations for larger amounts of adipose tissue (hips, stomachs.,.) are termed 'adipose depots.'

Atherosclerosis: this is a gradual occlusion (obstruction) of the arteries with deposits of smooth muscle cells, lipids, white blood cells and connective tissue. Also known as 'hardening of the arteries'. The process causes cumulative damage to artery walls, and blood flow is eventually restricted; this is most dangerous when it effects the blood supply to the heart. A great deal of research, past and current, has concentrated on the prevention of atherosclerosis, which has been flagged as the precursor to heart attacks.

Bile Acid: Bile acid, or just 'bile', is an emulsifying salt that is secreted by the gall bladder to enhance fat emulsion and digestion. People who have had their gall bladder removed cannot tolerate high-fat meals, and seem to tolerate short and medium chain saturated fats better than other sorts.

Catalyst: A catalyst is a material which causes or accelerates a chemical reaction without becoming part of the reaction product. Impurities present during the processing of oils can act as catalysts of the oxidation process, and metal catalysts are used to change fatty acids into trans fats.

Cholesterol: Cholesterol is the waxy, fat-like substance that occurs naturally in all parts of the body, especially in the walls of cells, where it serves a crucial role in maintaining proper levels of permeability and rigidity. It is also an anti-oxidant. Excess blood cholesterol is associated with arterial and heart damage, but the relationship between these is so complex that I'm afraid you'll just have to read Chapters 14-16 of the book to understand it!

Cholesterolemic: cholesterol-raising.

Chylomicrons: These are small protein containers full of lipids, which they carry from the intestinal walls to the liver for processing or to adipose tissue for storage.

Cis and *trans* : See *Geometric Isomerism*

Co-factors: In lipid nutrition, these are the nutrients, especially vitamins and minerals, that are necessary for the processing of fats into the specific forms our bodies need.

Cold pressed oils: These are oils produced with strict limitations on the amount of heat generated, in order to ensure minimal temperature-induced oxidation. They are pressed only once, slowly, and in a controlled environment that limits exposure to light and air. Authentic cold pressed oils will need to be refrigerated *and* consumed within about six weeks of the container being opened.

Conjugated fatty acids: A type of polyunsaturated fatty acid with two or more unsaturated carbon atoms but not separated by a saturated carbon atom as in the regular double bonded fatty acids. Conjugated linoleic acid is the most common and well-known conjugated fatty acid; it is believed to have anti-cancer, anti-atherosclerosis and immune-boosting effects, but most people consume it as a supplement because of its metabolism-boosting properties.

Coronary Artery Disease, (CAD): This disease is characterised by the narrowing of the arteries, as a result of plaque and atherosclerosis, to the point that the blood supply to the heart is compromised. CAD generally takes a long time to develop, though the process can take less time for some than others.

Coronary Heart Disease, (CHD): A wide variety of diseases are lumped under this catch-all category, which includes many problems that the heart might have as a muscle, many of them unrelated to arterial damage. CHD can be ischemia, a lack of blood supply to the heart, causing a local deficiency of oxygen. Or coronary heart disease can take the form of a myocardial infarction, which results in a localized death of part of the heart muscle. CHD can also be organic in nature. The heart muscle can experience inflammation, damage from viral or bacterial diseases, autoimmune reactions, genetic disorders, congenital disorders, or any disorder that disrupts the enzymes and proteins that effect cardiac function.

Desaturase system: refers to a set of processes in which enzymes known as 'desaturases' restructure fatty acids by removing hydrogen atoms. The two most important roles of these enzymes are in the production of oleic acid out of saturated stearic acid, in and achieving a crucial process in the processing of essential fatty acids (EFAs).

Diet-Heart Hypothesis: This is the general term used to lump together the conclusions of all the research relating high animal fat diets and high dietary cholesterol to increased 'risk' (not incidence) of coronary heart disease.

Eicosanoids: is a collective term referring to the derivatives of fatty acids which stimulate hormone-like responses on a cellular level. They are formed from essential fatty acids through the elongation and desaturation reactions. They are the inflammatory and anti–inflammatory reactors for cellular needs. Eicosanoids are the prostaglandins, prostocyclines, thromboxanes, and leukotrienes.

Enzymatic desaturase system: see *desaturase system*

Essential fatty acid (EFA): The collective term for those fats which the body cannot produce itself – such as through the *desaturase system.* They are alpha-linolenic acid (a form of omega-3 fatty acid) and linoleic acid (a form of omega-6). The body uses these as building blocks for other, longer chain fatty acids which are important in many aspects of health. Read chapters 11 and 12 again: it's important!

Fatty Acid: This is the general term for any specific fat molecule – the substances that are found in various combinations in dietary fats and oils. They all share the same basic structure: at the beginning, or 'alpha' end there is a standard glycerol structure of carbon, oxygen and hydrogen. Attached to this are three chains of carbon atoms, with a greater or lesser number of hydrogen atoms attached to them, The carbon chains can be different lengths, and the hydrogen atoms can be attached in different configurations; it is these differences that define the fatty acid and its role and effects within the body.

Fatty Streaks: These are a normal and natural thickening of the arteries as a result of a build-up of white blood cells under the arterial wall, and are found in populations throughout the world, from adolescence onwards. Fatty streaks are not a hardening, but a *thickening* of the weakened areas of the artery wall, which widens to accommodate the deposits.

Geometric Isomerism: Unsaturated fatty acids can exist in either the cis or trans configuration depending on which side of the carbon atom chain joined by the double bonds the hydrogen molecules are attached If hydrogen atoms are on the same of the double bond the configuration is cis. If the hydrogen atoms are on opposite sides of the double bond the configuration is trans. The melting point is higher for fats with a greater percentage of trans fatty acids.

HDL cholesterol: high density lipoprotein cholesterol is a suitcase that carries tissue cholesterol away from the site and back to the liver for resynthesis or excretion. High density lipoprotein fractions have more protein and less cholesterol in their suitcase. Sometimes misleadingly called 'good cholesterol'.

Hydrogenation: this is the process by which hydrogen atoms are pumped into liquid oils in the presence of a metal catalyst. The hydrogen atoms attach to carbon atoms, changing the fatty acid saturation point and therefore the metabolic process of the original fatty acid. Hydrogenation can be complete or partial.

Hypercholesterolemia: 'Hyper' means just what it implies; too much of something. And hypercholesterolemia refers to there being too much cholesterol in the blood, as a consequence of a hereditary condition that affects a certain proportion of the population across cultures and throughout the world. In hypercholesterolemia, the cholesterol receptors in the liver do not function properly, and people with this gene are indeed wise to monitor their blood cholesterol levels, which can become unnaturally, dangerously high.

Interesterification: interesterification is a process in which enzymes are used to alter the molecular structure of a vegetable oil, to give it the properties of a saturated fat. This is done by separating the triglyceride molecule into its components — a glycerol and 3 fatty acid strands — and then recombining them in various ways, depending on the uses for which they are intended. These are not 'trans fats', but just like trans fats, these products have a molecular structure that combines bits that the body recognises with bits that do not function as natural fats would – they are a synthetic, non-functional product masquerading as food.

LDL cholesterol: 'low density lipoprotein' cholesterol is a suitcase that carries the manufactured cholesterol from the liver to the tissue to be deposited for repair. In low-density lipoproteins there is more cholesterol in the suitcase than protein molecules.

Linoleic Acid: (LA) is an omega-6 polyunsaturated fatty acid with 18 carbons and two double bonds. LA is said to be essential as the body cannot manufacture it from other foods. It is a precursor to other fatty acids and eicosanoids that can only be found in complete form in fatty fish. Linoleic acid is responsible for promoting inflammatory responses. Commonly just called omega 6, or omega 6 EFA (essential fatty acid).

Linolenic Acid: (LNA) is an omega-3 polyunsaturated fatty acid with 18 carbons and three double bonds. LNA is essential as it cannot be manufactured in the body and must be acquired from food sources. It is plentiful in flaxseeds, flaxseed oil, walnuts and hemp oil. It is the precursor for the super long and unsaturated oils EPA – eicosapentanoic acid and DHA – docosahexaenoic acid which are found preformed in fatty fish. It induces anti-inflammatory responses. Commonly just called omega 3, or omega 3 EFA (essential fatty acid).

Lipid; lipid is the general term for a whole range of organic substances. Fats and the fatty acids that make them up are an important sub-category of lipids, and the term lipid is often simply used to refer to fats.

Lipid bi-layer: Is the thin membrane that surrounds all cells, and some structures within cells. It is made up of two layers of lipids – including various phospholipids and cholesterol. Its role is to control what substances enter and leave a cell or its components. The health of the lipid bi-layer is a crucial element of general health.

Lipoprotein: is a protein structure that carries lipids in the blood stream.

Micronutrients: these are the vitamins and minerals – and a few other nutritional odds and ends – that the body needs. They are used in their own right, or as catalysts and building blocks in the body's use of proteins, carbohydrates and fats. Even though they are needed in very small amounts, they are essential for good health. A balanced diet of natural food, that is healthy in its own right, should provide all the micronutrients the body needs.

Monounsaturated fatty acids: are fatty acids that have one double-bonded (unsaturated) carbon in the carbon chain, with all of the remainder being single-bonded. Olive, canola and peanut oils contain high proportions of monounsaturated fatty acids.

Oxidation: is a basic chemical reaction, in which the interaction of two different substances triggers the loss of an electron in one of them. Oxygen is one universal oxidant, and gave the reaction its name. In the world of fatty acids, oxidation refers to three processes. The first is the process by which mitochondria break down fats for fuel. The second is the deterioration through oxidation of fats and oils while they are processed, stored or cooked – through exposure to oxygen, metal catalysts, salts, heat and ultraviolet light. The third is the unwanted oxidation of fatty acids within the human body, which is implicated in a host of disease states.

Phospholipids: are lipid compounds made up of fatty acids and phosphates. The main use of phospholipids is in the lipid bilayer of cells. They have both hydrophilic (water soluble) and hydrophobic (water repelling/ lipid soluble) parts – which accounts for their ability to maintain the structure and integrity of cells. Also known as phosphatides.

Plaque: This is an accumulation on the blood vessel walls of cholesterol deposits, other fats, and general debris. Plaque serves a purpose, in that it thickens blood vessel walls as they deteriorate from use. These walls incur more damage with high blood pressure, excessive free radicals and age. As it is, we all have plaque build up – especially at the bends, twists, and turns of artery walls where the pressure and strain are greatest.

Polyunsaturated fatty acids: are fatty acids that contain two or more double bonds in their fatty acid chain. These are the healthful but unstable fatty acids found in in highest concentrations in flax and hemp oils, fish, and nuts. Always store them properly.

Refined oils: come from a solvent-based extraction process, and the oils will contain some residue from the solvents. They also go on to be further refined, through degumming, deodorizing and bleaching. There are no restrictions on the temperatures and pressures that can be used to produce refined oils, and their colour will vary from clear to white. They have no odour.

Saturated fatty acid: is a fatty acid with no double bonds. Its carbon
chains are completely saturated with hydrogen molecules. It will
generally be solid at room temperature. Animal fats, palm and coconut oils have high concentrations of saturated fats.

Trans and cis: See *Geometric Isomerism*

Trans fats: are unsaturated fatty acids in which hydrogen atoms are attached to the carbon bonds in 'trans' (opposing) fashion. There are
a few naturally occurring trans fats, but most are products of the food
industry. Since they have been linked to a host of health problems,
most especially arterial damage, and offer absolutely no positive
health benefits, they should simply not be eaten at all.

Triglyceride: the standard form that edible fatty acids take, They are molecules made up of three fatty acids attached to a glycerol backbone
of three carbons. Triglycerides are used by the body as fuel storage
in adipose tissue and for organ protection. Triglycerides vary in their
chain length and saturation to the fatty acids by hydrogen molecules.

Unrefined oils: are mechanically pressed oils that are first cooked, and
then pressed. There are few standards or guidelines concerning the
amount of heat and pressure used. Unrefined oils will be less intense
in colour than virgin oils but still retain a golden hue. They have virtually no aroma.

Unsaturated fats: see *polyunsaturated fatty acids* and *monounsaturated
fatty acids.*

Virgin unrefined oil: is mechanically pressed, according to strictly en-
forced standards regarding with heat and pressure, and only once.
Virgin pressed oils are golden, or green. They have a degree of opac-
ity, and a pleasant aroma. Virgin olive oil is the most readily available, but other virgin unrefined oils can be found as well, and are
always the best option when choosing an unsaturated oil.

RECOMMENDED READING
AND BIBLIOGRAPHY

Recommended Reading

Here are a few books that I think are particularly useful for the interested layperson. Some are more challenging than others – and I've tried to indicate their level of difficulty.

Mary G. Enig, Ph.D. , 2000 *Know Your Fats: The Complete Primer for Understanding the Nutrition of Fats, Oils, and Cholesterol.*
This book was written for the educated consumer. I think it offers a great summary of fats and oils. Another good addition to any health-conscious person's library but it might be a bit complex if you find yourself struggling with biochemistry.

· Mary Enig, MD. and Sally Fallon, 2005, *Eat Fat Lose Fat.*
Mary Enig is a renowned lipid biochemist whose complex research is expressed in a reader friendly manner by Sally Fallon. The two are a great team and they have collectively been able to simplify complex topics of nutrition. Their work is highly recommended for the beginner health reader.

Michael L. Gurr. 1999 *Lipids in Nutrition and Health: A Reappraisal.*
This is a wonderful, systematised book. Gurr's writing style lets him take very complex biochemistry topics and make them digestible for the enthusiastic health reader. His approach is scientific, in that it does not have an agenda; he simply presents the facts about research he cites, the

biochemistry of fats and how human health benefits from fats. I read the hard copy and it is my bible. A PDF version of the book is available at www.pjbarnes.co.uk/op/nutpdf.htm.

Uffe Ravnskov, MD, PhD., 2000 *The Cholesterol Myths, Exposing the Fallacy That Saturated Fat and CholesterolCause Heart Disease.*

Also a good summary of research that is often cited in research papers. Not a hard read, but take notes as you go and this will be a good resource for understanding your own blood profiles.

Eric Schlosser, 2004 *Fast Food Nation.*

Easy read that gives insight into the ill effects of mass processed foods – on our health, on the treatment of animals, the conditions of workers, and the health of the planet.

Ron Schmid, ND, 2003 *The Untold Story of Milk, Green Pastures, Contented Cows and Raw Dairy Foods.*

A very important book for understanding processing of all foods. It's centred on milk, but touches on many other issues as well, such as cholesterol, animal fats and heart disease, and the role of business and government in shaping our diets. Well written, easy to understand, and passionately opinionated.

Russell L. Smith Ph.D., with Edward R. Pinckney, MD, 1993 – *The Cholesterol Conspiracy.*

This is a recommended read for those looking to understand a bit more about the history of heart disease, and the politics behind the way that some diseases take centre stage while others are ignored.

Erasmus Udo, 1993 – *Fats that Heal, Fats that Kill.*

I have been following Udo for several decades now. He was really the researcher who brought omega 3 into the light and helped promote the idea of 'good fats.' I constantly use this as a resource, and I've read it several times cover to cover. It is meant to be for the general public but it can be pretty challenging; I know that some people who've read it have misinterpreted some of the chemistry. Still, it's a good addition to the library of any health conscious person. Read it in segments, carefully, and it will be very useful.

Other Sources

All the technical sections of the book are firmly based on existing science: here are the sources I used – available at a good university library.

Books

Armand B. Christophe and Stephanie DeVriese, editors, 2000, Fat Digestion and Absorption.

John M. DeMan, Ph.D., 1980, Principles of Food Chemistry.

N.A.M. Eskin, H.M.Henderson, R.J.Townsend, 1971, Biochemistry of Foods.

Edwin N. Frankel, 1998, Lipid Oxidation.

James L. Groff, Sareen S. Gropper, 2000 *Advanced Nutrition and Human Metabolism, Third Edition*, -

M.I. Gurr, J.L. Harwood, K.N. Frayn, 2002, Lipid Biochemistry, 5th Edition,

Yung-Sheng Huang, Shing-Jong Lin, Po-Chao Huang, Editors, 2003, Essential Fatty Acids and Eicosanoids, Invited Papers from the 5th International Congress,,

Afat Kamal-Eldin, Marjukka Makinen, Anna-Maija Lampi, The challenging contribution of hydroperoxides to the lipid oxidation mechanism In A. Kamal-Eldin ed. *Lipid oxidation pathways.*

Dharma R. Kodali and Gary R. List, Editors, 2005, Trans Fats Alternatives,

Gary R. List, David Kritchevsky, and Nimal Ratnayake, Editors 2007 Trans Fats In Foods.

Robert A. Moreau, Afaf Kamal-Eldin, Editors, 2009, Gourmet and Health-Promoting Specialty Oils.

Christopher D. Moyes, Patricia M. Schulte, 2008, Principles of Animal

Physiology, 2nd Edition,

Roman Przybylski and Bruce E. Macdonald, editors, 1995, Development and Processing of Vegetable Oils for Human Nutrition.

J.L. Sebedio and W.W. Christie, Editors, 1998, *Trans Fatty Acids in Human Nutrition.*

Jean-Louis Sebedio, William W. Christie, Richard Adlof, Editors, 2003, Advances in Conjugated Linoleic Acid Research, Vol.,2.

Lorraine P. Turcotte, Erik A. Richter and Bente Kiens, 2006, Exercise Metabolism, in Mark Hargreaves, editor, *Lipid Metabolism During Exercise.*

Erasmus Udo, Ph.D Fats and Oils, 1st edition,. 1986

Ronald R. Watson, Editor 2009 Fatty Acids in Health Promotion and Disease Causation.

Nedyalka V. Yanishlieva and Emma M. Marinova, 2003, Kinetic Evaluation of the Antioxidant Activity in Lipid Oxidation, pg. 85-107, in Afaf Kamal-Elidin, editor Lipid Oxidation Pathways.

Periodicals

Inform, International News on Fats, Oils, and Related Materials,

May 2009 Vol., 20 (5) 273-336, June 2009, Vol., 20(6) 337-400, December 2005, Vol., 16 (12) 725-788, January 2006, Vol., 19(1) 1-72, April 2007, Vol., 18 (4) 209-296, July 2006, vol., 17 (7) 401-488, June 2008, Vol., 19(6) 361-424, March 2007, Vol., 18(3), 145-208, March 2008, Vol., 19(3) 137-200, August 2005,Vol., 16(8) 473-536, January 2005, Vol., 16(1) 1-64, July 2007, Vol., 18 (17), 425-516, May 2006, Vol., 17(5), 273-336, June 2006, Vol., 17(6) 337-400, March 2006, Vol., 17(3), 129-192, Octorber 2006, Vol., 17(10), 617-680, April 2008, Vol., 19(4), 201-296, August 2006, Vol., 17(8) 489-552,

Food Product Design, Applications, Reinventing Oil Stability, Donna Berry, April 2007, 43-52

Canadian Meat Business, March/April, 2009, Vol., 8 Number 2

The Journal of Nutrition, Official Publication of the American Society for Nutritional Scicences, January 2000, Vol., 130(1), November 2000, Vol., 130(11), July 2000, Vol., 130(7), August 2000, Vol., 130(8S), August 2000, Vol., (8), February Vol., 130(2S)

Finally, here are a few internet sources of useful information

EFA (essential fatty acids) education, produced by The Polyunsaturated Fatty Acid Special Interest Group
http://efaeducation.nih.gov/

The Institute of Shortening and Edible Oils website.
www.iseo.org

A canola oil information website
www.canolainfo.org

FAO (Food and Agriculture Organisation) Fats and Oils in Human Nutrition
Chapter 1-10, April 5, 2007
http://www.fao.org/docrep/ V4700E/V4700E00.htm

The Weston A. Price Foundation, This is a good site for current health topics.
www.westonaprice.org

A website about coconut oil
http://www.coconut-info.com/

DHA/EPA Omega-3 Institute Science-based DHA/EPA Omega-3 Information
www.DHAomega3.org.